The Low FODMAP Protocol for Women Made Simple

Relieve Digestive Disorders and Manage IBS with a Tailored 60-Day Plan of Easy, Fast Meals on a Budget

Sarah Milton

Sarah Milton © Copyright 2024. All rights reserved.

The content contained within this book may not be reproduced, duplicated, or transmitted without direct written permission from the author or the publisher.

Under no circumstances will any blame or legal responsibility be held against the publisher, or author, for any damages, reparation, or monetary loss due to the information contained within this book, either directly or indirectly.

Legal Notice:

This book is copyright-protected. It is only for personal use. You cannot amend, distribute, sell, use, quote or paraphrase any part, or the content within this book, without the consent of the author or publisher.

Disclaimer Notice:

Please note the information contained within this document is for educational and entertainment purposes only. All effort has been executed to present accurate, up-to-date, reliable, and complete information. No warranties of any kind are declared or implied. Readers acknowledge that the author is not engaging in the rendering of legal, financial, medical or professional advice. The content within this book has been derived from various sources. Please consult a licensed professional before attempting any techniques outlined in this book.

By reading this document, the reader agrees that under no circumstances is the author responsible for any losses, direct or indirect, that are incurred as a result of the use of the information contained within this document, including, but not limited to, errors, omissions, or inaccuracies.

TABLE OF CONTENTS

INTRODUCTION 9

WHY THE LOW-FODMAP DIET? 9
UNDERSTANDING DIGESTIVE HEALTH IN WOMEN 9
IBS AND THE ROLE OF DIET 11
HOW TO USE THIS BOOK 13
OVERVIEW OF THE 60-DAY PLAN 13

PART I: UNDERSTANDING THE LOW-FODMAP DIET AND DIGESTIVE HEALTH ... 15

CHAPTER 1: WHAT ARE FODMAPS? 15

UNDERSTANDING FODMAPS: THE BASICS 15
BENEFITS OF A LOW-FODMAP DIET 16
COMMON DIGESTIVE DISORDERS: IBS, BLOATING, GAS, AND CRAMPING 16
HOW FODMAPS TRIGGER SYMPTOMS 17

CHAPTER 2: WOMEN'S DIGESTIVE HEALTH & HORMONAL INFLUENCE 19

HOW IBS AND DIGESTIVE ISSUES AFFECT WOMEN DIFFERENTLY 19
THE ROLE OF HORMONES IN GUT HEALTH 20
MANAGING SYMPTOMS DURING MENSTRUAL CYCLES, PREGNANCY, AND MENOPAUSE ... 21

CHAPTER 3: THE THREE PHASES OF THE LOW-FODMAP DIET 23

ELIMINATION PHASE: RESETTING THE DIGESTIVE SYSTEM (WEEKS 1-2) 23
REINTRODUCTION PHASE: IDENTIFYING TRIGGERS (WEEKS 3-5) 24
PERSONALIZATION PHASE: LONG-TERM MAINTENANCE (WEEKS 6-8) 25

CHAPTER 4: GETTING READY FOR THE LOW-FODMAP DIET 27

KITCHEN ESSENTIALS AND TOOLS FOR SUCCESS 27

| How to Read Labels for Hidden FODMAPs | 29 |

PART II: THE 60-DAY LOW-FODMAP PROTOCOL — 32

CHAPTER 5: ELIMINATION PHASE (DAYS 1-14) — 32

Goal: Reset Your Gut Health	32
Overview of Allowed and Avoided Foods	33
Sample Week 1 Meal Plan	33
Sample Week 2 Meal Plan (Breakfast, Lunch, Dinner, Snacks)	35

CHAPTER 6: REINTRODUCTION PHASE (DAYS 15-35) — 36

Goal: Identify Your Personal Triggers	36
How to Reintroduce Foods Safely	38
Sample Week 3-4-5 Meal Plans	40

CHAPTER 7: PERSONALIZATION PHASE (DAYS 36-60) — 43

| Sample Week 6-7-8 Meal Plans | 43 |
| Maintaining Digestive Health After the 60-Day Plan | 48 |

PART III: THE LOW-FODMAP RECIPE COLLECTION — 50

CHAPTER 8: BREAKFASTS ON A BUDGET — 51

Almond Butter Banana Overnight Oats	51
Almond Milk Chia Pudding	51
Blueberry Coconut Overnight Oats	52
Avocado Kiwi Bowl	52
Blueberry Spinach Smoothie	53
Chive and Cheddar Omelet	53
Cinnamon Walnut Overnight Oats	54
Cottage Cheese and Pineapple Bowl	54
Cucumber Kiwi Bowl	55

Cucumber Melon Smoothie	55
Egg and Avocado Breakfast Wrap	56
Gluten-Free Toast with Peanut Butter and Blueberries	56
Kiwi Pineapple Smoothie	57
Oatmeal with Almonds and Maple Syrup	57
Papaya Pineapple Smoothie	58
Peanut Butter Banana Smoothie	58
Pineapple Ginger Smoothie	59
Rice Cakes with Smoked Salmon and Cucumbers	59
Scrambled Eggs with Bell Peppers	60
Smoothie Bowl with Mango and Spinach	60
Spinach and Blueberry Smoothie Bowl	61
Spinach Mango Smoothie	61
Strawberry Almond Overnight Oats	62
Strawberry Orange Smoothie	62
Sweet Potato and Egg Scramble	63

CHAPTER 9 (25 RECIPES): FAST AND EASY LUNCHES   **64**

Avocado and Egg Salad Sandwich	64
Avocado and Tuna Salad	64
Brown Rice and Kale Bowl	65
Brown Rice and Roasted Carrot Bowl	65
Buckwheat and Zucchini Bowl	66
Buffalo Chicken Wrap	66
Caprese Wrap	67
Chicken and Rice Stir-Fry	67
Coconut Shrimp and Rice	68
Egg and Potato Salad	68
Ground Turkey and Sweet Potato Skillet	69
Ham and Spinach Sandwich	69
Hummus and Cucumber Wrap	70
Lentil and Carrot Stew	70
Millet and Grilled Zucchini Bowl	71

Millet and Roasted Eggplant Bowl	71
Quinoa and Roasted Vegetable Salad	72
Quinoa and Sweet Potato Bowl	72
Quinoa and Roasted Bell Pepper Bowl	73
Quinoa and Roasted Carrot Bowl	73
Rice and Stir-Fried Bok Choy Bowl	74
Rice and Turkey Lettuce Wraps	74
Spinach and Feta Scramble	75
Sweet Potato and Black Bean Bowl	75
Wild Rice and Roasted Bell Pepper Bowl	76

CHAPTER 10 (25 RECIPES): EFFORTLESS DINNERS — 77

Baked Lemon Chicken and Green Beans	77
Balsamic Glazed Salmon and Asparagus	77
Basil Pesto Quinoa	78
Beef and Bell Pepper Fajitas	78
Beef and Quinoa Skillet	79
Chicken and Sweet Potato Sheet Pan	79
Chicken and Zucchini Stir-Fry	80
Garlic-Infused Shrimp and Zucchini	80
Honey Mustard Chicken with Sweet Potatoes	81
Lemon Herb Chicken Pasta	81
Lemon Herb Tilapia and Broccoli	82
Lentil and Spinach Stew	82
One-Pot Lemon Chicken and Rice	83
Pasta with Roasted Red Pepper Sauce	83
Peanut Noodles	84
Pesto Rice with Grilled Chicken	84
Pork and Potato Hash	85
Rice with Tomato Basil Sauce	85
Roasted Chicken Sausage with Bell Peppers	86
Roasted Tofu with Brussels Sprouts	86
Salmon and Rice Bowl	87

SHRIMP AND LEMON RISOTTO	87
TOFU AND VEGETABLE STIR-FRY	88
TURKEY AND BELL PEPPER SKILLET	88
TURKEY AND ZUCCHINI MEATBALLS WITH ROASTED POTATOES	89

CHAPTER 11 (25 RECIPES): SNACKS AND ON-THE-GO SOLUTIONS — 90

ALMOND BUTTER RICE CAKES	90
BANANA COCONUT CHIA PUDDING	90
BANANA OAT MUFFINS	91
BLUEBERRY ALMOND GRANOLA BARS	91
BLUEBERRY ALMOND MUG CAKE	92
BLUEBERRY CHIA PUDDING	92
CINNAMON WALNUT OAT BARS	93
COCONUT ALMOND ENERGY BALLS	93
CUCUMBER AND TURKEY ROLL-UPS	94
DARK CHOCOLATE ALMOND ENERGY BARS	94
DARK CHOCOLATE DIPPED STRAWBERRIES	95
EGG SALAD LETTUCE CUPS	95
GLUTEN-FREE CRACKERS WITH AVOCADO SLICES	96
HARD-BOILED EGGS WITH CHERRY TOMATOES	96
HONEY ALMOND NUT MIX	97
KALE CHIPS	97
LACTOSE-FREE GREEK YOGURT PARFAIT	98
PEANUT BUTTER AND CELERY STICKS	98
PEANUT BUTTER CHOCOLATE CHIP COOKIES (GLUTEN-FREE)	99
PEANUT BUTTER OAT ENERGY BITES	99
RASPBERRY COCONUT MACAROONS	100
ROASTED PUMPKIN SEEDS	100
TURKEY AND SWISS LETTUCE WRAPS	101
ZUCCHINI CHIPS	101
WALNUT AND DATE ENERGY BITES	102

PART IV: EXPERT TIPS AND STRATEGIES FOR SUCCESS — 103

CHAPTER 14: MANAGING IBS AND DIGESTIVE ISSUES BEYOND DIET — 103

Stress Management and Its Role in Gut Health — 103
Sleep, Exercise, and Their Impact on Digestion — 104

CHAPTER 15: NAVIGATING SOCIAL EVENTS AND DINING OUT — 106

How to Stick to Low-FODMAP at Restaurants — 106
Tips for Traveling While Following the Diet — 107

CHAPTER 16: SUPPLEMENTS AND ADDITIONAL SUPPORT — 109

Probiotics, Prebiotics, and Their Role in Gut Health — 109
Supplements for IBS Management — 110

CONCLUSION — 112

Recap of the 60-Day Journey — 112
How to Maintain Long-Term Digestive Health — 112

INTRODUCTION

Welcome to the Low-FODMAP Protocol, a powerful tool designed to help you regain control of your digestive health. Whether you're struggling with IBS or other digestive discomforts, this book will guide you through a practical, science-based approach to reducing your symptoms and improving your quality of life. The Low-FODMAP diet isn't just another trend; it's a clinically proven method to manage the very real challenges that come with digestive disorders. My goal is to make this journey simple, manageable, and sustainable, so you can focus less on what's bothering your gut and more on living your life fully.

Why the Low-FODMAP Diet?

Understanding Digestive Health in Women

Understanding digestive health in women is a critical component of addressing and managing gut-related issues, especially when considering the Low-FODMAP diet. Women experience unique challenges when it comes to digestive health due to the intricate relationship between hormones, the gut, and overall wellbeing. Many digestive issues—such as irritable bowel syndrome (IBS)—disproportionately affect women, and understanding the underlying reasons for this can help you take better control of your health.

One of the key differences in digestive health between men and women is the impact of hormonal fluctuations. Hormones like estrogen and progesterone play a significant role in women's digestive function, and these hormones fluctuate throughout the menstrual cycle, during pregnancy, and later in life through menopause. These shifts can directly affect the way your gut functions, leading to changes in bowel movements, bloating, and even pain.

During the menstrual cycle, for example, many women report increased bloating, gas, or constipation as a result of hormonal shifts. Progesterone, in particular, can slow down bowel motility, leading to feelings of sluggish digestion or even constipation in the luteal phase (the time between ovulation and the start of your period). Meanwhile, lower estrogen levels can also contribute to gastrointestinal symptoms, affecting how your body processes foods and absorbs nutrients.

If you've experienced these fluctuations, it's not just a coincidence—your digestive system and hormones are deeply connected. Recognizing these patterns in your digestive health can help you make better dietary and lifestyle choices to mitigate symptoms. During certain phases of your cycle, you might find it helpful to adjust your intake of high-FODMAP foods or eat smaller, more frequent meals to avoid overwhelming your digestive system.

It's well-documented that IBS is more prevalent in women than in men, and it often manifests differently. Women with IBS may experience more severe constipation, bloating, or alternating between constipation and diarrhea, which are all exacerbated by hormonal changes.

For those of you who have IBS, you may have noticed that stress and emotional factors can worsen your symptoms. This is another area where the gut-brain connection plays a role. Women tend to report higher levels of stress and anxiety, which can have a direct impact on digestive health. The gut contains millions of neurons and is highly responsive to emotional states—this is often referred to as the "second brain." So, when stress levels are high, your gut may react by slowing down digestion, increasing sensitivity to discomfort, or even speeding up bowel movements.

Understanding this complex relationship between your brain and gut can empower you to manage your symptoms more effectively. Stress reduction techniques such as mindfulness, yoga, or even simple breathing exercises can help you take control of stress-related digestive symptoms.

Women also face digestive health challenges that evolve over different life stages. Pregnancy, for instance, brings dramatic changes to the body's digestive function. Many women experience heartburn, constipation, or bloating during pregnancy due to increased pressure on the digestive organs and the relaxation of muscles in the digestive tract caused by elevated levels of progesterone. In these moments, a Low-FODMAP approach may help reduce bloating and gas, but it's essential to adjust the diet in a way that ensures proper nutrition for both you and your growing baby.

Similarly, menopause brings its own set of challenges. As estrogen levels decline, digestive health may be impacted in new ways. Lower estrogen levels can lead to changes in gut motility, potentially causing new or exacerbated symptoms of IBS. For some women, this transition may mean revisiting and refining the Low-FODMAP diet to manage evolving symptoms.

Fiber is an essential nutrient for digestive health, and it's especially important for women, who are more prone to constipation, particularly as they age. However, fiber can be tricky for those following a Low-FODMAP diet. High-FODMAP foods like certain grains, legumes, and fruits are often rich in fiber, but they can also trigger digestive discomfort.

Finding a balance between getting enough fiber while avoiding trigger foods is key. Low-FODMAP, fiber-rich options such as chia seeds, oats, and kiwi are great alternatives that can help you maintain regular bowel movements without aggravating symptoms. Including a variety of these foods in your diet will support your gut health while ensuring you get the fiber you need to prevent constipation and support the beneficial bacteria in your gut.

The gut microbiota, or the community of bacteria living in your digestive tract, plays a critical role in overall digestive health. Women's microbiota can be influenced by many factors, including hormonal changes, diet, and antibiotic use. Maintaining a healthy microbiota through diverse, low-FODMAP foods and possibly including probiotic-rich foods like lactose-free yogurt can contribute to better digestion and fewer IBS symptoms.

Because every woman's body is different, there is no one-size-fits-all approach to maintaining digestive health. The beauty of the Low-FODMAP diet, particularly in the reintroduction and personalization phases, is that it allows you to identify which foods work for your unique body. As you move forward, it's important to continue paying attention to how your body responds to different foods and adjust your intake as needed.

By understanding the link between hormones, gut health, and life stages, you can approach your digestive health in a more informed and intuitive way. With this knowledge, you're equipped to make choices that enhance your overall wellbeing, keeping both your gut and your whole body in balance. In summary, digestive health in women is deeply intertwined with hormonal cycles, stress, and life stages. Recognizing these connections and taking a personalized, mindful approach to your diet and lifestyle will help you maintain long-term digestive wellness.

IBS and the Role of Diet

Irritable Bowel Syndrome (IBS) is a functional gastrointestinal disorder that affects how your gut works, causing symptoms like bloating, cramping, gas, and changes in bowel habits. Although it doesn't cause permanent damage to the intestines, the chronic discomfort and unpredictability of symptoms can significantly impact your quality of life. For many, the role of diet is crucial in managing IBS, and understanding how specific foods interact with your gut is key to finding relief.

Diet plays an integral role in both triggering and alleviating IBS symptoms. Certain foods can exacerbate the symptoms of IBS by causing fermentation in the gut, leading to gas, bloating, and discomfort. On the other hand, a well-planned, targeted approach to eating can calm the gut and help you regain control over your symptoms.

The Low-FODMAP diet has become one of the most well-researched and effective strategies for managing IBS. It targets a specific group of short-chain carbohydrates and sugars that are not fully absorbed in the gut. These fermentable oligosaccharides, disaccharides, monosaccharides, and polyols—collectively referred to as FODMAPs—can be difficult to digest and are known to trigger symptoms in people with IBS.

By reducing your intake of high-FODMAP foods and then systematically reintroducing them, you can identify which specific types of FODMAPs your gut is sensitive to and which foods you can tolerate without triggering symptoms. This process of elimination, reintroduction, and personalization allows you to maintain a broader, more balanced diet while avoiding your personal triggers.

When you consume foods high in FODMAPs, they travel to the small intestine, where they are poorly absorbed and continue into the large intestine. Here, they draw in water and are fermented by gut bacteria, producing gas as a byproduct. This fermentation and gas production can lead to bloating, cramping, and changes in bowel movements, whether it's diarrhea, constipation, or an alternating pattern of both.

The increased water in the gut can also lead to diarrhea by speeding up the transit of stool through the intestines. Conversely, if the fermentation process causes gas and bloating without expelling waste quickly, it may slow down motility, resulting in constipation. For many individuals with IBS, this creates a frustrating cycle of discomfort that can feel difficult to manage without clear dietary guidelines.

This is where the Low-FODMAP diet shines—it provides a structured way to control what goes into your gut and helps you understand how specific foods affect your digestive system.

Although diet is one of the most influential factors in managing IBS, it's important to recognize that other lifestyle factors also play a role. Stress, sleep, and physical activity can all influence gut function and exacerbate IBS symptoms.

The gut-brain connection is particularly relevant for those with IBS. Your digestive system contains millions of nerve cells that communicate directly with your brain, and stress or anxiety can significantly impact gut function. Many people with IBS notice a worsening of symptoms during periods of high stress. Incorporating stress management techniques—such as mindfulness, yoga, or breathing exercises—into your daily routine can improve your overall symptom control.

Physical activity also plays a role in maintaining digestive health. Gentle exercises, such as walking, yoga, or swimming, can stimulate bowel motility and help alleviate symptoms of constipation. Finding the right balance of activity for your body can further support the positive dietary changes you've implemented.

IBS is a chronic condition, but with the right tools, you can successfully manage your symptoms long-term. The Low-FODMAP diet provides a structured approach to identifying and managing food triggers, but it's only one piece of the puzzle. The key to long-term success is finding a balance between diet, stress management, and lifestyle adjustments that work for you.

You may find that as your body changes over time, so too do your triggers and tolerances. Being mindful of how your body responds to food and staying open to adjusting your diet accordingly can help you maintain better control over your IBS symptoms. Furthermore, engaging with a healthcare professional or dietitian who specializes in digestive health can provide additional support and guidance as you navigate this journey.

How to Use This Book

Overview of the 60-Day Plan

This book is designed to be your comprehensive guide to managing IBS and digestive discomfort through a structured Low-FODMAP diet. The 60-day plan it outlines provides a clear path toward understanding your personal food triggers and reclaiming control over your digestive health. Whether you're new to the Low-FODMAP diet or have tried it before, this approach will help you navigate the complexity of food sensitivities in a methodical and supportive way. Let's walk through how to best use this book and what you can expect over the next 60 days.

The structure of this book is intentional, starting with the foundational science behind FODMAPs and IBS, followed by practical meal plans and recipes tailored for each phase of the diet. The goal is not only to help you eliminate foods that may trigger symptoms but also to guide you in reintroducing them systematically, so you can identify your personal sensitivities.

You should treat this book as a toolkit. The first part provides essential background information on why and how the Low-FODMAP diet works, giving you the knowledge you need to make informed decisions. The second part offers detailed meal plans, complete with a wide variety of easy-to-make recipes. You'll find that these meals are designed to be both nourishing and enjoyable while sticking closely to the guidelines of the Low-FODMAP diet.

The 60-day plan is divided into three essential phases:

1. **Elimination Phase (Days 1–14)** – The focus of the first two weeks is on resetting your gut. During this phase, you will remove all high-FODMAP foods from your diet. By eliminating potential irritants, you'll give your digestive system a chance to rest and recover from the continuous strain of reactive foods. This phase might feel restrictive, but it's temporary and critical for establishing a baseline of symptom control.

2. **Reintroduction Phase (Days 15–35)** – Once you've experienced some relief in the elimination phase, you will move into the reintroduction phase. This is a crucial step where you will gradually test specific high-FODMAP foods in a controlled way, one at a time. The goal is to observe and record your body's reactions to each food group, identifying which types of FODMAPs cause symptoms and which you can tolerate. The process requires patience, as it's essential to reintroduce foods systematically to pinpoint the exact triggers.

3. **Personalization Phase (Days 36–60)** – After completing the reintroduction phase, you will have gathered valuable information about your food sensitivities. The personalization phase helps you apply that knowledge, adjusting your diet to include the foods that don't trigger symptoms while continuing to avoid those that do. This phase empowers you to build a long-term, sustainable eating plan that maximizes variety without compromising digestive comfort.

The meal plans and recipes provided in this book are designed to be flexible and adaptable. Whether you're someone who enjoys cooking from scratch or needs quick, on-the-go meal options, you'll find choices that fit your routine. The weekly meal plans offer suggestions for breakfast, lunch, dinner, and snacks, so you won't need to guess or feel overwhelmed about what to eat next.

Each recipe has been carefully crafted to ensure that it aligns with the principles of the Low-FODMAP diet while keeping in mind the importance of flavor, nutrition, and ease of preparation. You'll find that many of the meals use ingredients you likely already have on hand, making it easier to follow the plan without needing to drastically overhaul your pantry.

Keeping a food and symptom diary throughout the 60-day plan is vital for success. The ability to accurately track which foods cause symptoms will give you clear insights into your unique digestive responses. As you move through each phase, you'll be able to look back and make informed decisions based on data, rather than guessing. You may notice that while one food group is problematic, others are surprisingly well-tolerated. This information will form the basis of your personalized long-term eating plan.

PART I: UNDERSTANDING THE LOW-FODMAP DIET AND DIGESTIVE HEALTH

Part I of this book is your essential foundation for understanding the Low-FODMAP diet and how it can transform your digestive health. Whether you've been struggling with IBS or other gut-related issues, this section will guide you through the science behind FODMAPs—what they are, why they trigger symptoms, and how they affect your digestive system. You'll learn the key principles of the diet and how it can provide relief from the discomforts of bloating, gas, and cramping. By deepening your knowledge here, you'll be better equipped to manage your symptoms and start your journey toward a healthier, more balanced gut.

Chapter 1: What Are FODMAPs?

Understanding FODMAPs: The Basics

Understanding FODMAPs is essential to successfully managing your digestive health. FODMAPs, which stands for fermentable oligosaccharides, disaccharides, monosaccharides, and polyols, are short-chain carbohydrates that are poorly absorbed in the small intestine. These carbohydrates are found in many common foods, and for some of you, they can trigger uncomfortable digestive symptoms like bloating, gas, diarrhea, or constipation.

When FODMAPs aren't absorbed properly, they travel to the large intestine, where they ferment and draw water into the bowel. This fermentation process can lead to the overproduction of gas, which causes that feeling of fullness, pressure, and discomfort. Additionally, the excess water in the bowel can alter stool consistency, leading to diarrhea or, conversely, constipation in some cases.

The Low-FODMAP diet is designed to temporarily limit these triggering carbohydrates, giving your gut a chance to reset. During the Elimination Phase, you'll avoid high-FODMAP foods, allowing your symptoms to subside. By understanding how FODMAPs work within your digestive system, you'll have greater insight into why certain foods make you feel the way you do and how to take control of your gut health.

As you move forward, the goal is not to avoid FODMAPs forever, but to pinpoint which specific types cause you trouble. Through careful reintroduction, you'll be able to personalize your diet, maintain variety, and keep digestive symptoms at bay. The key is to strike a balance that works for your body while continuing to enjoy nourishing, satisfying meals.

Benefits of a Low-FODMAP Diet

The benefits of following a Low-FODMAP diet can be transformative, particularly for those of you managing IBS (Irritable Bowel Syndrome) or other functional gastrointestinal disorders. One of the most immediate advantages is the significant reduction in uncomfortable symptoms such as bloating, abdominal pain, gas, diarrhea, and constipation. By temporarily eliminating high-FODMAP foods, you allow your digestive system to calm down, reducing inflammation and irritation in the gut.

A well-structured Low-FODMAP diet helps you regain control over your digestive health. This diet empowers you to identify specific food triggers by reintroducing FODMAPs methodically after the Elimination Phase. It's not just about avoidance—it's about understanding how your body responds to various carbohydrates, so you can create a long-term, personalized eating plan.

Beyond symptom relief, there are psychological benefits as well. The unpredictability of digestive discomfort can affect your social life, work, and mental well-being. By controlling your symptoms, you'll likely experience improved mental clarity, energy, and a better quality of life overall. You can enjoy meals, travel, and social gatherings with greater confidence, knowing what your body can tolerate.

In addition, the Low-FODMAP diet promotes mindful eating. By being more conscious of your food choices, you'll likely develop a deeper connection to your health and nutrition. It can lead to healthier, more balanced eating habits even beyond the specific FODMAP guidelines.

Ultimately, the Low-FODMAP diet equips you with a clear understanding of your digestive system's needs, giving you the tools to maintain gut health long-term while still enjoying a varied and satisfying diet.

Common Digestive Disorders: IBS, Bloating, Gas, and Cramping

Common digestive disorders like IBS (Irritable Bowel Syndrome), bloating, gas, and cramping affect millions of people globally, and managing these conditions can feel overwhelming. Understanding the root causes of these symptoms is key to regaining control over your digestive health.

IBS is one of the most prevalent functional gastrointestinal disorders, characterized by chronic discomfort, irregular bowel movements, and often a heightened sensitivity to specific foods. Symptoms of IBS can vary widely from person to person, with some experiencing frequent bouts of diarrhea, while others struggle with constipation or alternating between both. Bloating, gas, and cramping are common companions to IBS, caused by the malabsorption of certain carbohydrates that ferment in the gut, leading to excessive gas production.

Bloating and gas, though uncomfortable, are often misunderstood. Bloating refers to the feeling of abdominal fullness or swelling, usually the result of trapped gas in the intestines. It can leave you feeling sluggish and self-conscious, especially after meals. Gas, on the other hand, is a natural byproduct of digestion, but excessive gas can cause discomfort and social anxiety. When it builds up too quickly or is not passed efficiently, it leads to cramping and pressure in the abdomen.

Cramping occurs when the muscles in the digestive tract contract too forcefully, often as a reaction to gut irritation or inflammation. This can be especially painful and is frequently associated with IBS flare-ups. For many, this cramping creates a cycle of anxiety and discomfort, further complicating the digestive process.

The Low-FODMAP diet is specifically designed to address these symptoms. FODMAPs (Fermentable Oligosaccharides, Disaccharides, Monosaccharides, and Polyols) are short-chain carbohydrates that are poorly absorbed in the small intestine. When they reach the colon, they ferment, producing gas and attracting water, leading to bloating, cramping, and irregular bowel movements. By eliminating high-FODMAP foods and carefully reintroducing them, you can identify which carbohydrates trigger your symptoms, allowing you to manage these digestive disorders with greater precision.

If you've been living with the frustration of IBS, bloating, gas, or cramping, understanding the role that FODMAPs play in your symptoms can be a game-changer. It gives you a practical approach to reducing or eliminating discomfort and improving your overall quality of life.

How FODMAPs Trigger Symptoms

When FODMAPs trigger symptoms, it all begins in the digestive tract. FODMAPs are a group of carbohydrates that are not well absorbed in the small intestine. For some of you, your gut doesn't break these down efficiently, allowing them to travel into the large intestine. Once there, two processes occur that lead to symptoms: fermentation by gut bacteria and an osmotic effect that draws water into the intestine.

First, the fermentation process is key. Gut bacteria feed on the unabsorbed FODMAPs, producing gases like hydrogen, methane, and carbon dioxide as byproducts. For many of you, this rapid gas production can cause significant bloating, cramping, and even pain, especially if your gut is more sensitive. This is why bloating and gas are often the most noticeable symptoms when you consume high-FODMAP foods.

Second, the osmotic effect is equally disruptive. Because FODMAPs attract water into the intestine, it can lead to diarrhea or loose stools for some individuals. The excess water disrupts the consistency and movement of stool, making digestion irregular. For others, this process can instead lead to constipation, as the imbalance between gas production and water absorption causes slower movement in the intestines.

What makes FODMAPs particularly tricky is their variability. Not all high-FODMAP foods will affect you in the same way, and each of you may react differently to specific types of FODMAPs. For example, lactose may cause severe symptoms for one person, while fructans or polyols might be the culprit for someone else. The type of FODMAP, the amount consumed, and your overall gut sensitivity combine to influence how your digestive system reacts.

By understanding how these compounds behave in your digestive system, you'll have a better grasp of why symptoms flare up when you eat certain foods. This is also why the reintroduction phase of the Low-FODMAP diet is so crucial. By systematically testing different FODMAP categories, you can identify which foods trigger your symptoms and to what extent. Armed with this knowledge, you'll be able to modify your diet in a way that supports your digestive health, without unnecessary restrictions.

Chapter 2: Women's Digestive Health & Hormonal Influence

How IBS and Digestive Issues Affect Women Differently

IBS and digestive issues affect women differently, and understanding these differences is essential for effective management, especially when considering a Low-FODMAP approach. Research shows that women are more likely to be diagnosed with IBS, and their symptoms can be influenced by a variety of factors, including hormonal fluctuations, psychological stress, and differences in gut motility. One of the most significant factors in how IBS affects women differently is the menstrual cycle. Hormonal changes, particularly fluctuations in estrogen and progesterone, play a role in modulating gut function. During certain phases of the menstrual cycle, particularly just before menstruation, many of you may notice an increase in IBS symptoms such as bloating, abdominal pain, and changes in bowel movements. This sensitivity is often tied to how hormones influence the digestive system's motility and the brain-gut connection, making symptom management more complex.

Additionally, studies suggest that women tend to experience more constipation-predominant IBS (IBS-C) than men. This may be linked to differences in gut motility, which tends to be slower in women, leading to a higher risk of constipation. On the other hand, stress can exacerbate IBS symptoms, and given that women often report higher levels of stress and anxiety, this psychological component can intensify the impact of IBS on daily life. The connection between stress and gut health, often referred to as the gut-brain axis, is a crucial aspect of managing digestive symptoms effectively.

IBS can also affect women's overall quality of life more intensely than it does for men. For many of you, the unpredictability of symptoms—bloating, gas, cramps—can disrupt work, social life, and even relationships. It's important to recognize this emotional and social toll when navigating your diet and health strategies. This is why a personalized approach, such as the Low-FODMAP diet, can be particularly beneficial. By understanding how your body reacts to different foods and external stressors, you can tailor your diet to alleviate symptoms while maintaining a balanced, fulfilling lifestyle.

Finally, reproductive health conditions like endometriosis and polycystic ovary syndrome (PCOS) can overlap with IBS symptoms, making it more challenging to distinguish between the two. Many of you may find that managing these coexisting conditions requires an even more thoughtful approach to diet and symptom tracking.

By recognizing how these factors interplay with digestive health, you can take a more holistic approach to managing IBS as a woman. The Low-FODMAP diet serves as a powerful tool to reduce symptom triggers, but it's also important to stay mindful of the broader context of your health—hormones, stress, and overall well-being—to successfully manage and improve your digestive health.

The Role of Hormones in Gut Health

Hormones play a significant role in gut health, especially for women, and understanding their impact is crucial for managing conditions like IBS and other digestive disorders. Hormones regulate many aspects of your body, and when it comes to gut function, their influence can be profound. In particular, fluctuations in estrogen and progesterone—key hormones involved in the menstrual cycle—can affect everything from bowel movements to gut motility and even the sensitivity of your digestive system.

Estrogen tends to have a protective effect on the gut lining, promoting a healthy gut barrier and influencing how your intestines absorb nutrients and process waste. However, as estrogen levels fluctuate during different phases of the menstrual cycle, this can lead to changes in digestion. For example, high estrogen levels can slow down gut motility, leading to bloating and constipation, while lower levels may contribute to faster motility, often associated with diarrhea.

Progesterone, on the other hand, is known for its slowing effect on the digestive system. During the luteal phase of your menstrual cycle, when progesterone peaks, you may notice a sluggish digestive system, which can increase feelings of fullness, bloating, and constipation. This is why many women experience digestive discomfort in the days leading up to their period. The rise in progesterone relaxes the smooth muscle in your intestines, which can make bowel movements slower and more difficult.

Beyond the menstrual cycle, other hormonal changes, such as those experienced during pregnancy or menopause, can further affect gut health. During pregnancy, for example, the combination of increased progesterone and pressure from the growing uterus can lead to common digestive issues like heartburn, constipation, and bloating. Similarly, during menopause, the drop in estrogen can weaken the protective function of the gut lining, potentially increasing sensitivity to foods and triggering IBS-like symptoms.

The connection between your gut and hormones isn't just limited to estrogen and progesterone. The stress hormone cortisol also plays a significant role in gut health. When you are stressed, your body releases cortisol, which can disrupt normal gut function by slowing down digestion or, conversely, speeding it up. This is one reason why stress is such a major trigger for IBS symptoms. Managing stress through mindfulness, relaxation techniques, and a healthy diet can help mitigate its impact on your digestive system.

Given this strong interplay between hormones and gut health, it becomes clear why many of you might experience heightened digestive symptoms at certain times of the month or during different life stages. By understanding how these hormonal changes affect your digestion, you can take a more proactive approach to managing your symptoms. The Low-FODMAP diet can help stabilize digestive issues during these hormonal fluctuations by reducing the intake of fermentable carbohydrates that might otherwise exacerbate symptoms during sensitive times.

Incorporating lifestyle strategies to balance your hormones, such as regular physical activity, stress management, and consuming a nutrient-dense diet, is essential to supporting your overall digestive health. Recognizing how your hormones impact your gut is a vital step in maintaining long-term well-being, especially as you fine-tune your Low-FODMAP plan to match your body's unique needs.

Managing Symptoms During Menstrual Cycles, Pregnancy, and Menopause

Managing digestive symptoms during different life stages—such as the menstrual cycle, pregnancy, and menopause—requires understanding how your body changes and how it affects your gut health. Each of these stages brings unique challenges, particularly for those managing conditions like IBS or other digestive sensitivities. By tuning into your body and using a structured approach like the Low-FODMAP diet, you can help reduce symptoms and maintain balance throughout these fluctuations.

Menstrual Cycle

During your menstrual cycle, fluctuations in hormones, particularly estrogen and progesterone, can significantly affect gut function. Many women notice increased bloating, gas, or changes in bowel habits—such as constipation or diarrhea—around their period. For example, high progesterone during the luteal phase can slow digestion, causing constipation, while the drop in progesterone just before menstruation may trigger diarrhea. These hormonal shifts can intensify IBS symptoms, making this time of the month especially challenging.

To manage these symptoms, it's important to stay consistent with your Low-FODMAP eating plan, which helps minimize foods that are more likely to cause gas, bloating, and discomfort. You may also want to focus on hydrating well, incorporating gentle forms of movement like yoga or walking, and choosing easily digestible meals during this time. Some find that eating smaller, more frequent meals helps prevent the bloating and discomfort that often accompany hormonal shifts.

Pregnancy

Pregnancy brings its own set of digestive challenges, with hormones like progesterone rising dramatically to support the pregnancy. This hormone relaxes the muscles of the digestive tract, often leading to slower digestion, constipation, and bloating. Additionally, the growing uterus can press on the stomach and intestines, exacerbating these symptoms. Heartburn and indigestion also become more common as pregnancy progresses.

During pregnancy, it's essential to maintain balanced nutrition while adjusting your diet to alleviate discomfort. While the Low-FODMAP diet can still be used safely during pregnancy, it's important to ensure you're getting enough fiber, fluids, and essential nutrients for both you and your baby. You may need to adjust portion sizes, eat smaller meals more frequently, and choose low-FODMAP fiber sources like oats, quinoa, and certain vegetables to help with constipation. Staying active with safe prenatal exercises and drinking plenty of water can also support better digestion.

Be mindful of certain high-FODMAP foods that can aggravate pregnancy-related digestive symptoms, such as garlic, onions, and certain dairy products. If nausea is an issue, bland, low-FODMAP options like rice cakes, gluten-free toast, or plain oatmeal can help. Remember, it's always best to consult with your healthcare provider to ensure you're meeting your nutritional needs while managing symptoms.

Menopause

As you enter menopause, the significant drop in estrogen levels can affect your gut health. Estrogen has a protective role in maintaining gut motility and lining integrity, and when levels decline, many women experience increased bloating, gas, and changes in bowel regularity. Additionally, stress during menopause—whether from hormonal imbalances or life changes—can exacerbate digestive symptoms, as stress directly affects gut function.

In this phase, managing digestive health becomes a balance of continuing your Low-FODMAP diet while also focusing on foods that support hormonal health. High-fiber, low-FODMAP foods can be particularly beneficial during menopause, as they can help counteract constipation while maintaining a stable gut environment. Additionally, incorporating foods rich in calcium and vitamin D is crucial during menopause to support bone health, but be cautious with dairy if lactose is a trigger for you.

Reducing stress through relaxation techniques, meditation, or even low-impact exercise like swimming or tai chi can be particularly helpful in managing both hormonal changes and digestive symptoms. This phase may also call for adjustments in portion sizes and meal timing, as your metabolism slows with age, and large meals can feel more taxing on your digestive system.

Chapter 3: The Three Phases of the Low-FODMAP Diet

Elimination Phase: Resetting the Digestive System (Weeks 1-2)

The Elimination Phase is the foundation of the Low-FODMAP diet, designed to reset your digestive system and bring relief from the symptoms associated with IBS and other functional gastrointestinal disorders. During these first two weeks, your goal is to remove all high-FODMAP foods from your diet. This strict elimination allows your gut to heal and reduces the fermentable carbohydrates that often lead to bloating, gas, abdominal pain, and irregular bowel movements.

In this phase, you'll follow a carefully structured plan focused on low-FODMAP foods. These foods are less likely to trigger digestive distress because they don't ferment as much in the gut, which means less gas production, less water retention in the intestines, and, ultimately, less discomfort. Think of this phase as a reset button for your digestive system—removing the foods that overwhelm your gut so it can begin to function more smoothly.

While the process may seem restrictive at first, the simplicity of the elimination phase provides a clear roadmap: stick to low-FODMAP foods consistently for the duration of these two weeks. This allows your digestive system the chance to calm down, creating a baseline to identify which foods are truly causing your symptoms. You may notice that your symptoms improve within a few days, but it's important to complete the full two weeks for maximum benefit.

Some key aspects to remember during this phase:

- **Consistency is critical**: Every meal and snack should adhere to low-FODMAP guidelines. Even small amounts of high-FODMAP foods can trigger symptoms, so adherence is crucial.
- **Variety within limits**: While you'll be avoiding high-FODMAP foods, there's still plenty of variety to keep meals satisfying. Focus on lean proteins, low-FODMAP vegetables, gluten-free grains, and lactose-free dairy alternatives. You'll find plenty of delicious options within these categories.
- **Mind your portions**: Even low-FODMAP foods can trigger symptoms if eaten in excess. The FODMAP load can build up, so paying attention to recommended portion sizes is essential during this phase.

Additionally, keep track of your symptoms. Record how your body feels day to day in a journal, noting any changes in symptoms, bowel habits, or overall digestion. This will be invaluable in the reintroduction phase when you begin testing high-FODMAP foods to identify your personal triggers.

The elimination phase is not about depriving yourself—it's about providing your body the opportunity to reset, to breathe, and to regain balance. It can be a period of empowerment, where you start to regain control over your digestive health. And by the end of this phase, you'll be well-prepared to move forward into the next step of the Low-FODMAP journey: reintroducing foods and discovering what works best for your unique digestive system.

Reintroduction Phase: Identifying Triggers (Weeks 3-5)

The Reintroduction Phase, spanning Weeks 3 to 5, is where the real discovery begins. After completing the Elimination Phase, your gut has had time to reset, and by now, you should be experiencing noticeable symptom relief. The next step is carefully reintroducing high-FODMAP foods into your diet to identify your specific triggers. This phase is crucial in personalizing your Low-FODMAP journey and gaining deeper insight into what your body tolerates best.

The reintroduction process follows a structured and methodical approach. Each food group of FODMAPs—fructose, lactose, polyols, fructans, and galacto-oligosaccharides (GOS)—is reintroduced one at a time. This allows you to isolate the impact of each type of FODMAP on your digestive system, so you can determine which specific groups or foods are causing discomfort.

Here's how it works:

1. **Choose a FODMAP group**: Start by selecting a food from one FODMAP group, such as fructose (for example, apples). Introduce this food in a controlled portion and observe how your body responds.
2. **Test in stages**: On Day 1, consume a small portion of the test food. Monitor your symptoms for 24 hours, then increase the portion slightly on Day 2 if no symptoms arise. Continue this process for three days. If symptoms appear at any point, you can stop and note this food or FODMAP group as a potential trigger.
3. **Observe and record**: Keep a detailed symptom journal throughout this phase. Track how your body reacts to each food, noting changes in bloating, gas, pain, or bowel habits. By tracking these responses, you'll build a comprehensive picture of your specific triggers.
4. **Take breaks between tests**: After testing a food or FODMAP group, return to your baseline Low-FODMAP diet for a few days to allow your symptoms to stabilize before moving on to the next food. This ensures that each reintroduction is evaluated independently.

The key here is patience and precision. It can be tempting to rush through this process, especially if you're eager to expand your food options, but taking your time will yield much more accurate and valuable results. Since different people can react differently to the same FODMAPs, personal triggers will vary. For example, one person might tolerate lactose without any issues, while another experiences discomfort even with small amounts of dairy.

This phase is about understanding your body's unique tolerances. Perhaps you discover that you can handle certain high-FODMAP foods in small portions but react to larger quantities. Or maybe you'll find that certain groups, like fructans or polyols, cause significant discomfort and need to be minimized in your long-term diet. The reintroduction phase equips you with the knowledge you need to manage your symptoms with confidence and flexibility moving forward.

By the end of this phase, you will have identified your personal "red flags" and safe zones when it comes to FODMAPs, giving you the freedom to make informed food choices without the constant worry of unexpected digestive flare-ups. This newfound understanding sets the stage for the personalization phase, where you'll fine-tune your diet based on the insights you've gained.

Personalization Phase: Long-term Maintenance (Weeks 6-8)

The Personalization Phase, covering Weeks 6 to 8, is where you begin to tailor the Low-FODMAP diet to your unique digestive needs, armed with the insights gained during the Reintroduction Phase. By now, you should have a clear sense of which FODMAPs trigger symptoms for you and which foods you can safely enjoy. This phase is about fine-tuning your approach to create a sustainable, long-term diet that keeps you feeling your best.

Long-term maintenance on a Low-FODMAP diet doesn't mean lifelong restriction. Instead, it's about balance and flexibility. During this phase, your goal is to integrate foods that you can tolerate in moderation, while minimizing or avoiding those that consistently trigger symptoms. Since everyone's tolerance is different, this period is key to creating a personalized approach that supports both your digestive health and overall well-being.

Key Principles of the Personalization Phase:

1. **Reintroducing variety**: Now that you've identified your personal triggers, it's time to bring back more variety to your meals. This helps prevent monotony in your diet and ensures you get a wide range of nutrients. Start reintroducing low- and moderate-FODMAP foods that you've identified as safe, while keeping high-FODMAP foods that trigger symptoms in smaller quantities or reserved for special occasions.

2. **Portion control**: For some foods, the quantity makes all the difference. You might find that while a small portion of a high-FODMAP food is well-tolerated, larger amounts lead to discomfort. In this phase, you'll get comfortable with managing portion sizes to enjoy a more varied diet without compromising your digestive health.

3. **Planning for flexibility**: Life is unpredictable, and you won't always have control over what's on your plate. During the Personalization Phase, it's important to build strategies for dining out, social events, and travel that allow you to stick to your FODMAP-friendly plan without stress. This could

mean carrying safe snacks, communicating your dietary needs to restaurant staff, or opting for low-FODMAP options when uncertainty arises.

4. **Addressing occasional flare-ups**: Even with careful planning, occasional digestive flare-ups may still occur. Understanding how to handle these situations is key to long-term success. You might return to a stricter low-FODMAP diet temporarily to calm symptoms, then gradually reintroduce foods as you regain stability. Learning to manage these fluctuations with confidence is part of mastering your long-term digestive health.

5. **Ongoing adjustments**: Your digestive system can change over time. As you progress through this phase, remain open to continuing to adjust your diet. For instance, a food that was initially well-tolerated may cause discomfort later, or vice versa. Stay mindful of how your body responds to new circumstances, such as stress or hormonal shifts, and adjust your food choices accordingly.

Throughout this Personalization Phase, listen to your body's signals. The ultimate goal is to craft a lifestyle that balances your personal food preferences, nutrition, and symptom management, empowering you to live symptom-free without feeling overly restricted. At the end of these eight weeks, you'll have a clear, personalized roadmap for maintaining your digestive health over the long term. This final phase isn't about rigid rules—it's about giving you control and confidence in your relationship with food.

Chapter 4: Getting Ready for the Low-FODMAP Diet

Kitchen Essentials and Tools for Success

To thrive on a Low-FODMAP diet, having a well-equipped kitchen is crucial. The right tools can help simplify meal preparation, save time, and ensure that your meals are not only nutritious but also delicious. Below are the essential kitchen items that will support your journey, from the elimination phase to long-term maintenance.

1. Non-Stick Cookware

Investing in high-quality non-stick pots and pans is a game changer. These allow you to cook with minimal oil, which is particularly useful when preparing lighter, gut-friendly meals. Non-stick surfaces also make cleaning easier, ensuring that meal prep doesn't turn into a chore. A sturdy non-stick skillet is essential for preparing quick, Low-FODMAP meals like scrambled eggs, sautéed vegetables, or seared meats.

2. Sharp Knives and a Cutting Board

A reliable set of knives and a good cutting board are fundamental tools in any kitchen. Prepping fresh, Low-FODMAP vegetables and fruits is a major part of this diet, so having sharp knives will speed up the process and reduce frustration. A sturdy wooden or plastic cutting board will protect your counters and make chopping, slicing, and dicing safer and more efficient.

3. Blender or Food Processor

As you'll frequently prepare smoothies, soups, sauces, and dips, a high-quality blender or food processor is invaluable. These appliances make it easy to create Low-FODMAP smoothie bowls, purées, and dressings. Whether you're blending up a spinach and blueberry smoothie or making your own pesto sauce, a reliable blender or processor ensures smooth textures and helps you create meals quickly.

4. Pressure Cooker or Instant Pot

A pressure cooker or Instant Pot can save you significant time, especially when preparing one-pot meals. It's perfect for making large batches of Low-FODMAP soups, stews, and grains like rice or quinoa. These devices are versatile, allowing you to sauté, slow-cook, or steam your meals with minimal effort, which can be a lifesaver on busy days.

5. Food Storage Containers

Meal prepping is key for staying on track with the Low-FODMAP diet, and having a variety of storage containers will make this process smoother. Choose durable, leak-proof, and BPA-free containers that are microwave and freezer-friendly. This allows you to portion out meals for the week, store snacks, or even freeze extras for a later date, ensuring you always have a Low-FODMAP option ready to go.

6. Spiralizer

A spiralizer can add variety and fun to your meals, helping you turn Low-FODMAP vegetables like zucchini, carrots, and cucumbers into noodle alternatives. Zucchini noodles, for instance, are an excellent substitute for traditional pasta, allowing you to enjoy your favorite dishes without triggering symptoms. Having a spiralizer helps you experiment with textures and keeps your meals interesting.

7. Garlic Infuser and Garlic-Infused Oil

Since garlic is high in FODMAPs but its flavor is often missed, a garlic-infuser or ready-made garlic-infused oil can be a valuable tool. Infusing oil with garlic provides the aroma and taste without the high-FODMAP content. Using this in place of raw garlic allows you to retain flavor in dishes like stir-fries, pasta sauces, and roasted vegetables, without compromising digestive health.

8. Digital Kitchen Scale

A digital kitchen scale is essential during the reintroduction and personalization phases when portion control is important. By accurately weighing ingredients, you can stay within your personal tolerance levels for moderate FODMAP foods. This tool helps you test your reactions to different amounts of food, making it easier to pinpoint triggers without guesswork.

9. Steamer Basket

Steaming is one of the healthiest ways to prepare Low-FODMAP vegetables, preserving their nutrients without adding extra fat or oil. A simple steamer basket is affordable and fits into most pots, allowing you to steam vegetables like spinach, carrots, or zucchini quickly. Steamed veggies can be the base for many dishes or a simple side to complement your meals.

10. Measuring Cups and Spoons

Precision is key when following a Low-FODMAP diet, particularly in the early phases. Having a set of measuring cups and spoons ensures you're accurately following recipes and consuming appropriate serving sizes. Many FODMAP foods are tolerable in specific amounts, so these tools help you keep track of what you're eating without triggering symptoms.

11. Reusable Silicone Bags

For environmentally-conscious meal prep and snack storage, reusable silicone bags are a great alternative to plastic. These are perfect for storing cut fruits, veggies, and portioned snacks. They can be frozen, microwaved, and used on-the-go, ensuring that you always have safe, Low-FODMAP snacks ready when hunger strikes.

How to Read Labels for Hidden FODMAPs

Reading food labels is an essential skill when following a Low-FODMAP diet. Many foods contain hidden sources of high-FODMAP ingredients that can trigger symptoms, even in seemingly safe products. Understanding how to scan labels and spot potential problem ingredients allows you to make informed decisions and avoid unnecessary digestive distress.

1. Start with the Ingredients List

When evaluating a packaged food, always begin with the ingredients list. High-FODMAP foods often hide in the form of additives, preservatives, or sweeteners. You'll need to familiarize yourself with common FODMAP-containing ingredients such as fructose, inulin, high-fructose corn syrup, honey, wheat, and certain types of sugar alcohols like sorbitol and mannitol.

Pay particular attention to the order of ingredients listed. Ingredients are listed in descending order by weight, so if a high-FODMAP ingredient appears at the top of the list, it means the product contains a significant amount. Conversely, if it's near the bottom, the amount might be smaller, but it's still worth noting depending on your sensitivity.

2. Watch for Hidden Sweeteners

Many packaged foods, especially snacks, sauces, and beverages, contain hidden FODMAPs in the form of sweeteners. Ingredients such as honey, agave syrup, and high-fructose corn syrup are high in fructose, a common trigger. Additionally, sugar alcohols like sorbitol, xylitol, and mannitol are often used as low-calorie sweeteners in sugar-free products, but they are high in FODMAPs and can lead to bloating and gas.

Always be cautious with products labeled "sugar-free" or "diet," as these often use sugar alcohols to replace sugar. While they may seem like a healthier option, they are often problematic for those managing digestive issues.

3. Be Aware of Fructans and Galactooligosaccharides (GOS)

Fructans and GOS are two types of FODMAPs commonly found in certain grains, vegetables, and legumes. Wheat, rye, onions, and garlic are major sources of fructans, while GOS can be found in beans and lentils. The challenge is that even small amounts of garlic or onion powder can be added to many processed foods, including sauces, soups, dressings, and marinades, making it easy to overlook.

Look for terms such as "onion powder," "garlic powder," or "hydrolyzed vegetable protein" on ingredient labels. These often signal the presence of high-FODMAP foods. Even though these ingredients might be in tiny amounts, if you're in the elimination or early reintroduction phase, it's better to avoid them to prevent triggering symptoms.

4. Identify Problematic Fibers

While fiber is generally healthy and beneficial for digestion, some types of fiber are high in FODMAPs and can cause issues. Inulin and chicory root are commonly added to boost fiber content in products like granola bars, cereal, and yogurt, but they are both high in fructans. These can easily slip into foods marketed as "high-fiber" or "gut-friendly," so it's crucial to read labels carefully.

If you see "inulin," "chicory root extract," or "oligosaccharides" listed on a product, proceed with caution. These fibers can be problematic even in small amounts.

5. Check for Dairy Derivatives

Lactose, a common FODMAP, is present in many dairy products, but it can also be hidden in less obvious foods. Beyond milk, cream, and yogurt, lactose can be found in processed foods like baked goods, salad dressings, and even certain breads. Labels that list ingredients like "milk solids," "whey," or "milk powder" may indicate the presence of lactose.

If you're sensitive to lactose, look for products labeled "lactose-free" or those that use alternative ingredients like lactose-free milk, almond milk, or coconut milk. These alternatives will help you avoid digestive discomfort without sacrificing taste or texture.

6. Understanding Serving Sizes and Thresholds

Some FODMAPs are only problematic in larger quantities, so understanding serving sizes is key. For example, certain foods like almonds or avocado are considered moderate FODMAP foods. A small amount might be well-tolerated, but exceeding the threshold could trigger symptoms. Pay attention to serving sizes on packaging and compare them to recommended Low-FODMAP portions to stay within your personal tolerance.

When purchasing packaged foods, you may come across ingredients that are generally high-FODMAP but could be present in small amounts. For instance, a product with a tiny amount of honey may still be safe depending on the overall serving size. Your reintroduction phase will give you insights into which thresholds work for you.

7. Gluten-Free Does Not Always Mean Low-FODMAP

While many people on a Low-FODMAP diet avoid gluten-containing foods, it's important to note that gluten and FODMAPs are not synonymous. Gluten-free products can still contain high-FODMAP ingredients like honey, onion, garlic, or certain types of beans. Just because something is labeled "gluten-free" doesn't mean it's automatically Low-FODMAP.

Always check the full ingredient list rather than relying solely on marketing labels like "gluten-free" or "organic." This ensures you avoid any hidden FODMAP triggers that might lurk in seemingly safe products.

8. Use Low-FODMAP Certification as a Guide

To make shopping easier, some products now carry Low-FODMAP certification. This label ensures that the food has been tested and meets strict guidelines to be classified as Low-FODMAP. While this label is a helpful shortcut, not all products will carry it. For those that do, it can save you time and worry when selecting processed foods.

Using certified products can be particularly helpful in the elimination phase when strict adherence to Low-FODMAP foods is critical for resetting your gut and identifying triggers.

PART II: THE 60-DAY LOW-FODMAP PROTOCOL

Embarking on the 60-day Low-FODMAP protocol is an essential step toward understanding your body's unique triggers and finding long-term relief from digestive discomfort. This phase is more than just eliminating certain foods—it's a structured journey that guides you through discovery, reintroduction, and personalization, helping you reclaim control over your diet and well-being. Over the next two months, you'll move through three key phases: elimination, reintroduction, and personalization. Each phase is designed to fine-tune your understanding of what your body can tolerate, empowering you to make informed choices that suit your lifestyle and support lasting digestive health.

Chapter 5: Elimination Phase (Days 1-14)

Goal: Reset Your Gut Health

The elimination phase is a critical first step in resetting your digestive system and identifying the foods that may be triggering your symptoms. During these first 14 days, your goal is to drastically reduce the intake of high-FODMAP foods that may be fermenting in the gut and causing discomfort, such as bloating, gas, and cramping. This phase acts as a clean slate, allowing your gut to heal and reducing inflammation.

By eliminating FODMAPs, you give your digestive system the break it needs, offering immediate relief from symptoms while preparing the groundwork for the next steps in understanding your unique food sensitivities. These two weeks can feel restrictive, but they are crucial to gaining insight into how your body reacts to certain foods. The key is to stay consistent, focus on the allowed low-FODMAP foods, and embrace simple, nourishing meals that will support your gut reset.

This phase is not about deprivation—it's about empowerment. As you progress, you'll begin to notice subtle changes in how your body feels and responds, giving you the foundation to reintroduce foods confidently in the next stage of the protocol.

Overview of Allowed and Avoided Foods

During the elimination phase, knowing exactly which foods to include and which to avoid is essential for success. This period is designed to minimize the intake of high-FODMAP foods that can ferment in your gut and cause irritation, allowing your digestive system to reset. While it may seem restrictive at first glance, there are still plenty of delicious and nourishing options to choose from.

Allowed Foods include those low in FODMAPs, which are easier on your digestive system. You can enjoy a variety of lean proteins like chicken, turkey, and fish. Eggs are a great source of protein, as are firm tofu and lactose-free dairy products. Most leafy greens and low-FODMAP vegetables such as spinach, carrots, cucumbers, and bell peppers can be included without worry. Fruits like strawberries, blueberries, kiwis, and oranges are excellent choices, offering sweetness without the high FODMAP content. Grains such as gluten-free oats, quinoa, rice, and gluten-free bread are safe to consume, while herbs, spices, and garlic-infused oils can add flavor without triggering symptoms.

Avoided Foods consist of those that are high in FODMAPs, which can ferment and cause digestive distress. These include certain fruits like apples, pears, watermelon, and stone fruits, which are higher in fructose. Vegetables such as onions, garlic, cauliflower, and mushrooms are also off-limits due to their oligosaccharide content. Legumes like lentils and chickpeas (in large amounts), dairy products containing lactose, and wheat-based products like bread, pasta, and cereals should be avoided. Sweeteners such as high-fructose corn syrup, honey, and sugar alcohols are also high-FODMAP culprits.

Sticking to the allowed foods may feel limiting at first, but it's the key to helping your gut heal and reducing inflammation. These two weeks are a short-term investment in your long-term digestive health, and once the elimination phase is complete, you'll begin reintroducing foods with greater clarity about what your body can tolerate.

Sample Week 1 Meal Plan

To support your digestive reset during the elimination phase, this 7-day meal plan focuses on variety and simplicity using only low-FODMAP foods. The plan balances nourishing meals with enjoyable snacks to help you stay satisfied while reducing symptoms. You can rotate these meals and snacks throughout the week based on your needs, ensuring each day feels fresh and enjoyable.

Day 1
Breakfast: Almond Butter Banana Overnight Oats
Morning Snack: Almond Butter Rice Cakes
Lunch: Quinoa and Sweet Potato Bowl
Afternoon Snack: Hard-Boiled Eggs with Cherry Tomatoes
Dinner: Baked Lemon Chicken and Green Beans

Day 2

Breakfast: Blueberry Spinach Smoothie

Morning Snack: Coconut Almond Energy Balls

Lunch: Avocado and Egg Salad Sandwich

Afternoon Snack: Kale Chips

Dinner: Beef and Quinoa Skillet

Day 3

Breakfast: Chive and Cheddar Omelet

Morning Snack: Peanut Butter Oat Energy Bites

Lunch: Lentil and Spinach Stew

Afternoon Snack: Gluten-Free Crackers with Avocado Slices

Dinner: Lemon Herb Tilapia and Broccoli

Day 4

Breakfast: Strawberry Orange Smoothie

Morning Snack: Blueberry Almond Granola Bars

Lunch: Chicken and Rice Stir-Fry

Afternoon Snack: Dark Chocolate Almond Energy Bars

Dinner: Garlic-Infused Shrimp and Zucchini

Day 5

Breakfast: Cottage Cheese and Pineapple Bowl

Morning Snack: Zucchini Chips

Lunch: Buffalo Chicken Wrap

Afternoon Snack: Banana Coconut Chia Pudding

Dinner: Turkey and Bell Pepper Skillet

Day 6

Breakfast: Spinach Mango Smoothie

Morning Snack: Egg Salad Lettuce Cups

Lunch: Caprese Wrap

Afternoon Snack: Roasted Pumpkin Seeds

Dinner: Roasted Chicken Sausage with Bell Peppers

Day 7

Breakfast: Cinnamon Walnut Overnight Oats

Morning Snack: Cucumber and Turkey Roll-Ups

Lunch: Rice and Turkey Lettuce Wraps

Afternoon Snack: Blueberry Chia Pudding

Dinner: Tofu and Vegetable Stir-Fry

Sample Week 2 Meal Plan (Breakfast, Lunch, Dinner, Snacks)

This meal plan is tailored for Week 2 of the elimination phase, focusing on nourishing, low-FODMAP meals and snacks that support your gut health. Each day provides variety, while using familiar, budget-friendly ingredients to keep your meals enjoyable.

Day 1
Breakfast: Almond Butter Banana Overnight Oats
Morning Snack: Peanut Butter and Celery Sticks
Lunch: Avocado and Tuna Salad
Afternoon Snack: Hard-Boiled Eggs with Cherry Tomatoes
Dinner: Baked Lemon Chicken and Green Beans

Day 2
Breakfast: Blueberry Spinach Smoothie
Morning Snack: Coconut Almond Energy Balls
Lunch: Quinoa and Roasted Vegetable Salad
Afternoon Snack: Zucchini Chips
Dinner: Beef and Bell Pepper Fajitas

Day 3
Breakfast: Chive and Cheddar Omelet
Morning Snack: Almond Butter Rice Cakes
Lunch: Chicken and Rice Stir-Fry
Afternoon Snack: Gluten-Free Crackers with Avocado Slices
Dinner: Lemon Herb Tilapia and Broccoli

Day 4
Breakfast: Strawberry Almond Overnight Oats
Morning Snack: Cucumber and Turkey Roll-Ups
Lunch: Lentil and Carrot Stew
Afternoon Snack: Roasted Pumpkin Seeds
Dinner: Shrimp and Lemon Risotto

Day 5
Breakfast: Cottage Cheese and Pineapple Bowl
Morning Snack: Peanut Butter Oat Energy Bites
Lunch: Brown Rice and Kale Bowl
Afternoon Snack: Kale Chips
Dinner: Honey Mustard Chicken with Sweet Potatoes

Day 6
Breakfast: Cucumber Kiwi Bowl
Morning Snack: Banana Coconut Chia Pudding
Lunch: Hummus and Cucumber Wrap
Afternoon Snack: Blueberry Chia Pudding
Dinner: Turkey and Bell Pepper Skillet

Day 7
Breakfast: Cinnamon Walnut Overnight Oats
Morning Snack: Dark Chocolate Dipped Strawberries
Lunch: Egg and Potato Salad
Afternoon Snack: Lactose-Free Greek Yogurt Parfait
Dinner: Roasted Chicken Sausage with Bell Peppers

Chapter 6: Reintroduction Phase (Days 15-35)

Goal: Identify Your Personal Triggers

The ultimate goal of the reintroduction phase is to identify your personal triggers—specific FODMAP groups or foods that cause digestive symptoms for you. This phase is essential because it allows you to move from the initial restrictive elimination phase to a more sustainable, personalized diet, providing long-term relief without unnecessary restrictions. You're not meant to stay on a fully low-FODMAP diet indefinitely; instead, this phase is your opportunity to understand your unique thresholds and sensitivities, guiding you toward a balanced and enjoyable way of eating.

Each of us has a unique digestive response to FODMAPs. While certain FODMAP groups may trigger symptoms for one person, another person may tolerate them well. The reintroduction phase provides clarity by helping you determine which FODMAPs you can include in your diet and in what amounts. This knowledge empowers you to manage your symptoms with precision and flexibility.

To identify these triggers, you will systematically reintroduce one FODMAP group at a time into your diet. For example, you might start with lactose-containing foods for three to four days, gradually increasing the portion sizes while carefully monitoring any symptoms. After testing each FODMAP group, you'll return to the baseline low-FODMAP diet for a few days to allow your body to reset before introducing the next group. This step-by-step approach ensures that you can pinpoint exactly which foods cause issues and at what quantity.

The reintroduction phase requires patience and attention to detail. Rushing through it or testing multiple FODMAPs at once can blur the results and leave you uncertain about which foods are problematic. Consistency in tracking symptoms, food portions, and FODMAP groups is crucial for drawing clear conclusions. This is where a symptom journal becomes invaluable—you can record not only what you eat, but also how you feel, allowing you to see patterns over time.

Recognizing Symptom Patterns

Symptoms to look out for include bloating, gas, abdominal pain, diarrhea, and constipation. Each of these symptoms can be triggered by different FODMAPs. For example, you might experience bloating with foods high in fructans (like onions or garlic) but have no issues with lactose-containing dairy products. Identifying such patterns will help you fine-tune your diet in a way that's specific to your body's needs.

During this phase, you might also notice that certain foods are well tolerated in small amounts but trigger symptoms when eaten in larger portions. This insight allows you to personalize your diet not just by what you eat, but also by how much you can comfortably consume. For instance, while you may be able to enjoy a small portion of apples (high in fructose), a larger serving might cause discomfort. These nuances are important for creating a flexible diet that maximizes variety without causing symptoms.

Once you've completed the reintroduction phase and identified your personal triggers, your diet becomes more flexible. While some FODMAP groups or foods might need to be avoided entirely, others can be reintroduced in moderate amounts, offering you more freedom in your daily eating habits. The personalization of your diet is about balance—finding what works best for your body while still enjoying a variety of foods.

For example, you might discover that you can tolerate small amounts of wheat bread or yogurt, which allows you to include these items in your meals without discomfort. Or you may learn that garlic is a strong trigger, meaning you'll need to continue using garlic-infused oil as a substitute to avoid symptoms. This knowledge will help you navigate social events, dining out, and everyday meals with confidence and clarity, reducing the anxiety that often accompanies IBS and food intolerances.

Identifying your personal triggers doesn't just improve your physical well-being—it also reduces the mental strain of worrying about food. Once you've gone through the process and gained insight into what works for you, you'll feel more in control. The reintroduction phase is empowering because it gives you the tools to manage your symptoms proactively rather than reactively.

It's common to feel a sense of relief and newfound confidence when you understand your body's unique responses. Instead of living in fear of a random flare-up, you can take control by making informed choices that work for you. As you navigate this phase, you're not only identifying triggers but also building a sustainable and healthy relationship with food.

At the end of the reintroduction phase, you will have established a solid foundation for long-term gut health. The knowledge you gain during this time will support you in maintaining a balanced and diverse diet that meets your nutritional needs without triggering uncomfortable symptoms. You'll no longer need to rely on guesswork, as you'll have clear insights into which foods to include, avoid, or moderate.

The goal of this phase is to equip you with the skills and understanding needed to maintain your digestive health over the long term, without the burden of unnecessary restrictions. You will be able to enjoy meals with more confidence and less anxiety, knowing what works for your body and what doesn't. By identifying your personal FODMAP triggers, you're taking a major step toward a more comfortable, fulfilling life with food.

How to Reintroduce Foods Safely

Reintroducing foods safely during the reintroduction phase of the Low-FODMAP diet is crucial for identifying which specific FODMAP groups or foods trigger your digestive symptoms. To do this effectively, you'll need to take a systematic and careful approach, ensuring that you can clearly observe your body's reactions. This process will allow you to expand your diet beyond the elimination phase while still managing symptoms effectively. Below is a detailed guide on how to reintroduce foods safely.

1. **Step 1: Introduce One FODMAP Group at a Time**

The key to success in the reintroduction phase is testing one FODMAP group at a time. This will help you clearly identify which category of FODMAPs triggers symptoms. The main FODMAP groups are:

- **Fructose** (e.g., honey, apples, pears)
- **Lactose** (e.g., milk, soft cheeses, yogurt)
- **Fructans** (e.g., onions, garlic, wheat products)
- **Galactans** (e.g., beans, lentils, chickpeas)
- **Polyols** (e.g., stone fruits like peaches and cherries, sweeteners like sorbitol)

Start by selecting one group to reintroduce, and then test different foods from that group across multiple days.

2. **Step 2: Choose Your Test Foods**

Select one food from the FODMAP group you're testing. Choose a food that's high in the particular FODMAP but doesn't contain significant amounts of other FODMAPs, so you can accurately assess your reaction. For example:

- For **fructose**, test foods like honey or apples.
- For **lactose**, test milk or soft cheese.
- For **fructans**, test foods like garlic or wheat bread.
- For **galactans**, test lentils or chickpeas.
- For **polyols**, test stone fruits like peaches or sweeteners like sorbitol.

3. **Step 3: Start with a Small Portion**

Begin with a very small portion of the chosen food. For example, you might start with one teaspoon of honey, a small slice of bread, or a few pieces of apple. The goal is to test your tolerance gradually, starting with a small amount that's less likely to trigger a severe reaction.

4. **Step 4: Increase the Portion Over Several Days**

If no symptoms occur after the first small portion, gradually increase the amount over three days. For example:

- **Day 1**: Start with a small portion (e.g., 1 teaspoon of honey).
- **Day 2**: If no symptoms occur, increase to a moderate portion (e.g., 2 teaspoons of honey).
- **Day 3**: Increase to a regular portion (e.g., 1 tablespoon of honey).

This gradual increase will help you identify the threshold at which symptoms begin, allowing you to fine-tune your intake of that particular food.

5. **Step 5: Monitor and Record Symptoms**

Throughout the reintroduction process, keep a detailed food and symptom diary. Record:

- The food and portion size you ate
- Any digestive symptoms that occur (e.g., bloating, gas, cramping, diarrhea, constipation)
- The timing of the symptoms (e.g., immediately after eating, 2 hours later)

By tracking your symptoms, you'll begin to see patterns and determine how your body responds to specific FODMAPs. This will help you establish your personal tolerance levels.

6. **Step 6: Return to the Elimination Diet Between Tests**

After testing each food for 3-4 days, return to the elimination phase diet for a few days before moving on to the next FODMAP group. This "washout period" ensures that any symptoms from the previous test have fully subsided before you introduce the next food. It helps to reset your digestive system and prevents confusion between reactions from different FODMAP groups.

7. **Step 7: Repeat the Process for Each FODMAP Group**

After completing the washout period, move on to the next FODMAP group and repeat the process. Continue testing one group at a time, following the same steps of starting small, increasing the portion, monitoring symptoms, and taking a washout period between tests.

8. **Step 8: Note Tolerance Thresholds**

For some FODMAPs, you may find that you can tolerate small amounts but develop symptoms with larger portions. For example, you might be able to eat a small amount of wheat bread without issues but experience bloating after a larger portion. Noting these thresholds allows you to personalize your diet. You may not need to completely eliminate a particular FODMAP—just moderate the quantity.

9. **Step 9: Be Aware of Cumulative Effects**

Some FODMAPs have cumulative effects, meaning you might tolerate small amounts of multiple FODMAPs in isolation, but consuming several high-FODMAP foods together could trigger symptoms.

This is why it's important to reintroduce foods one at a time and remain mindful of how your body responds to combinations in the future.

10. Step 10: Adjust Based on Your Findings

At the end of the reintroduction phase, you'll have a much clearer understanding of which FODMAPs you tolerate well, which you can have in moderation, and which are best avoided altogether. With this knowledge, you can reintroduce a wide range of foods into your diet while keeping symptom triggers at bay.

11. Additional Tips for Success

- **Stay patient**: The reintroduction phase requires time and attention, but it's worth the effort for the insights it provides. Rushing this phase can lead to confusing results.
- **Work with a dietitian if needed**: If you're unsure about any aspect of reintroducing foods or need help navigating your symptoms, consider working with a dietitian who specializes in FODMAPs and IBS.
- **Be flexible**: Your tolerance levels may change over time, depending on factors like stress, illness, or overall gut health. Reassess your triggers periodically if necessary.

Sample Week 3-4-5 Meal Plans

The reintroduction phase is an essential part of the Low-FODMAP journey. During this period, you'll gradually test specific FODMAPs while maintaining balance and nourishment. The meal plan below is designed to support this testing process, helping you track your reactions while still enjoying variety and flexibility in your meals. You'll continue with low-FODMAP meals while adding back specific foods as per your reintroduction schedule.

Day 1
Breakfast: Almond Butter Banana Overnight Oats
Morning Snack: Zucchini Chips
Lunch: Avocado and Tuna Salad
Afternoon Snack: Peanut Butter Oat Energy Bites
Dinner: Chicken and Zucchini Stir-Fry

Day 2

Breakfast: Kiwi Pineapple Smoothie

Morning Snack: Dark Chocolate Dipped Strawberries

Lunch: Brown Rice and Roasted Carrot Bowl

Afternoon Snack: Almond Butter Rice Cakes

Dinner: Garlic-Infused Shrimp and Zucchini

Day 3

Breakfast: Blueberry Spinach Smoothie

Morning Snack: Cucumber and Turkey Roll-Ups

Lunch: Egg and Potato Salad

Afternoon Snack: Kale Chips

Dinner: Baked Lemon Chicken and Green Beans

Day 4

Breakfast: Cinnamon Walnut Overnight Oats

Morning Snack: Coconut Almond Energy Balls

Lunch: Quinoa and Roasted Vegetable Salad

Afternoon Snack: Hard-Boiled Eggs with Cherry Tomatoes

Dinner: Honey Mustard Chicken with Sweet Potatoes

Day 5

Breakfast: Almond Milk Chia Pudding

Morning Snack: Peanut Butter and Celery Sticks

Lunch: Chicken and Rice Stir-Fry

Afternoon Snack: Roasted Pumpkin Seeds

Dinner: Beef and Quinoa Skillet

Day 6

Breakfast: Cottage Cheese and Pineapple Bowl

Morning Snack: Blueberry Almond Granola Bars

Lunch: Buffalo Chicken Wrap

Afternoon Snack: Raspberry Coconut Macaroons

Dinner: Salmon and Rice Bowl

Day 7

Breakfast: Egg and Avocado Breakfast Wrap

Morning Snack: Blueberry Chia Pudding

Lunch: Quinoa and Sweet Potato Bowl

Afternoon Snack: Walnut and Date Energy Bites

Dinner: Pork and Potato Hash

Day 8

Breakfast: Papaya Pineapple Smoothie

Morning Snack: Gluten-Free Crackers with Avocado Slices

Lunch: Caprese Wrap

Afternoon Snack: Peanut Butter Chocolate Chip Cookies (Gluten-Free)

Dinner: Turkey and Bell Pepper Skillet

Day 9

Breakfast: Scrambled Eggs with Bell Peppers

Morning Snack: Honey Almond Nut Mix

Lunch: Lentil and Carrot Stew

Afternoon Snack: Dark Chocolate Almond Energy Bars

Dinner: One-Pot Lemon Chicken and Rice

Day 10

Breakfast: Avocado Kiwi Bowl

Morning Snack: Cucumber Kiwi Bowl
Lunch: Rice and Stir-Fried Bok Choy Bowl
Afternoon Snack: Banana Oat Muffins
Dinner: Lemon Herb Tilapia and Broccoli

Morning Snack: Kale Chips
Lunch: Hummus and Cucumber Wrap
Afternoon Snack: Dark Chocolate Dipped Strawberries
Dinner: Beef and Bell Pepper Fajitas

Day 11
Breakfast: Peanut Butter Banana Smoothie
Morning Snack: Peanut Butter Oat Energy Bites
Lunch: Avocado and Egg Salad Sandwich
Afternoon Snack: Zucchini Chips
Dinner: Roasted Tofu with Brussels Sprouts

Day 12
Breakfast: Strawberry Almond Overnight Oats
Morning Snack: Coconut Almond Energy Balls
Lunch: Ground Turkey and Sweet Potato Skillet
Afternoon Snack: Raspberry Coconut Macaroons
Dinner: Pasta with Roasted Red Pepper Sauce

Day 13
Breakfast: Pineapple Ginger Smoothie
Morning Snack: Blueberry Almond Mug Cake
Lunch: Brown Rice and Kale Bowl
Afternoon Snack: Hard-Boiled Eggs with Cherry Tomatoes
Dinner: Shrimp and Lemon Risotto

Day 14
Breakfast: Spinach Mango Smoothie

Day 15
Breakfast: Chive and Cheddar Omelet
Morning Snack: Cucumber and Turkey Roll-Ups
Lunch: Quinoa and Roasted Bell Pepper Bowl
Afternoon Snack: Blueberry Chia Pudding
Dinner: Chicken and Sweet Potato Sheet Pan

Day 16
Breakfast: Cucumber Melon Smoothie
Morning Snack: Dark Chocolate Almond Energy Bars
Lunch: Brown Rice and Roasted Carrot Bowl
Afternoon Snack: Peanut Butter and Celery Sticks
Dinner: Garlic-Infused Shrimp and Zucchini

Day 17
Breakfast: Almond Butter Banana Overnight Oats
Morning Snack: Zucchini Chips
Lunch: Chicken and Rice Stir-Fry
Afternoon Snack: Peanut Butter Chocolate Chip Cookies (Gluten-Free)
Dinner: Honey Mustard Chicken with Sweet Potatoes

Day 18

Breakfast: Spinach and Blueberry Smoothie Bowl
Morning Snack: Hard-Boiled Eggs with Cherry Tomatoes
Lunch: Egg and Potato Salad
Afternoon Snack: Coconut Almond Energy Balls
Dinner: Beef and Quinoa Skillet

Day 19

Breakfast: Oatmeal with Almonds and Maple Syrup
Morning Snack: Kale Chips
Lunch: Hummus and Cucumber Wrap
Afternoon Snack: Walnut and Date Energy Bites
Dinner: Salmon and Rice Bowl

Day 20

Breakfast: Strawberry Orange Smoothie
Morning Snack: Peanut Butter Oat Energy Bites
Lunch: Quinoa and Roasted Vegetable Salad
Afternoon Snack: Dark Chocolate Dipped Strawberries
Dinner: Turkey and Bell Pepper Skillet

Day 21

Breakfast: Cottage Cheese and Pineapple Bowl
Morning Snack: Blueberry Almond Granola Bars
Lunch: Rice and Turkey Lettuce Wraps
Afternoon Snack: Banana Coconut Chia Pudding
Dinner: Shrimp and Lemon Risotto

Chapter 7: Personalization Phase (Days 36-60)

Sample Week 6-7-8 Meal Plans

In this phase, you'll tailor your meals to the knowledge you've gained from the reintroduction phase, focusing on personal triggers and maintaining digestive balance. This 24-day meal plan provides diverse, satisfying Low-FODMAP options while allowing room to reintroduce and test certain foods to fit your individual digestive health. Each day includes breakfast, two snacks, lunch, and dinner, all chosen from the rich variety of recipes provided.

Day 1

Breakfast: Almond Butter Banana Overnight Oats

Morning Snack: Kale Chips
Lunch: Quinoa and Roasted Vegetable Salad
Afternoon Snack: Coconut Almond Energy Balls
Dinner: Garlic-Infused Shrimp and Zucchini

Day 2
Breakfast: Cottage Cheese and Pineapple Bowl
Morning Snack: Walnut and Date Energy Bites
Lunch: Avocado and Tuna Salad
Afternoon Snack: Dark Chocolate Dipped Strawberries
Dinner: Lemon Herb Chicken Pasta

Day 3
Breakfast: Spinach and Blueberry Smoothie Bowl
Morning Snack: Peanut Butter Oat Energy Bites
Lunch: Brown Rice and Roasted Carrot Bowl
Afternoon Snack: Hard-Boiled Eggs with Cherry Tomatoes
Dinner: Beef and Bell Pepper Fajitas

Day 4
Breakfast: Blueberry Coconut Overnight Oats
Morning Snack: Zucchini Chips
Lunch: Chicken and Rice Stir-Fry
Afternoon Snack: Blueberry Almond Granola Bars
Dinner: Balsamic Glazed Salmon and Asparagus

Day 5
Breakfast: Papaya Pineapple Smoothie

Morning Snack: Gluten-Free Crackers with Avocado Slices
Lunch: Sweet Potato and Black Bean Bowl
Afternoon Snack: Peanut Butter and Celery Sticks
Dinner: Turkey and Zucchini Meatballs with Roasted Potatoes

Day 6
Breakfast: Chive and Cheddar Omelet
Morning Snack: Almond Butter Rice Cakes
Lunch: Hummus and Cucumber Wrap
Afternoon Snack: Blueberry Chia Pudding
Dinner: One-Pot Lemon Chicken and Rice

Day 7
Breakfast: Kiwi Pineapple Smoothie
Morning Snack: Cucumber and Turkey Roll-Ups
Lunch: Millet and Grilled Zucchini Bowl
Afternoon Snack: Peanut Butter Chocolate Chip Cookies (Gluten-Free)
Dinner: Shrimp and Lemon Risotto

Day 8
Breakfast: Almond Milk Chia Pudding
Morning Snack: Raspberry Coconut Macaroons
Lunch: Spinach and Feta Scramble
Afternoon Snack: Roasted Pumpkin Seeds
Dinner: Chicken and Zucchini Stir-Fry

Day 9

Breakfast: Scrambled Eggs with Bell Peppers
Morning Snack: Dark Chocolate Almond Energy Bars
Lunch: Buckwheat and Zucchini Bowl
Afternoon Snack: Kale Chips
Dinner: Basil Pesto Quinoa with Grilled Chicken

Day 10

Breakfast: Avocado Kiwi Bowl
Morning Snack: Egg Salad Lettuce Cups
Lunch: Brown Rice and Kale Bowl
Afternoon Snack: Honey Almond Nut Mix
Dinner: Baked Lemon Chicken and Green Beans

Day 11

Breakfast: Peanut Butter Banana Smoothie
Morning Snack: Peanut Butter Oat Energy Bites
Lunch: Rice and Turkey Lettuce Wraps
Afternoon Snack: Blueberry Almond Mug Cake
Dinner: Roasted Chicken Sausage with Bell Peppers

Day 12

Breakfast: Strawberry Almond Overnight Oats
Morning Snack: Hard-Boiled Eggs with Cherry Tomatoes
Lunch: Caprese Wrap
Afternoon Snack: Almond Butter Rice Cakes
Dinner: Lentil and Spinach Stew

Day 13

Breakfast: Pineapple Ginger Smoothie
Morning Snack: Cucumber and Turkey Roll-Ups
Lunch: Ground Turkey and Sweet Potato Skillet
Afternoon Snack: Coconut Almond Energy Balls
Dinner: Pork and Potato Hash

Day 14

Breakfast: Smoothie Bowl with Mango and Spinach
Morning Snack: Walnut and Date Energy Bites
Lunch: Quinoa and Sweet Potato Bowl
Afternoon Snack: Dark Chocolate Dipped Strawberries
Dinner: Salmon and Rice Bowl

Day 15

Breakfast: Oatmeal with Almonds and Maple Syrup
Morning Snack: Zucchini Chips
Lunch: Egg and Potato Salad
Afternoon Snack: Peanut Butter Chocolate Chip Cookies (Gluten-Free)
Dinner: Beef and Quinoa Skillet

Day 16

Breakfast: Blueberry Spinach Smoothie
Morning Snack: Blueberry Almond Granola Bars
Lunch: Quinoa and Roasted Bell Pepper Bowl
Afternoon Snack: Kale Chips

Dinner: Honey Mustard Chicken with Sweet Potatoes

Day 17
Breakfast: Almond Butter Banana Overnight Oats
Morning Snack: Dark Chocolate Almond Energy Bars
Lunch: Avocado and Egg Salad Sandwich
Afternoon Snack: Raspberry Coconut Macaroons
Dinner: Tofu and Vegetable Stir-Fry

Day 18
Breakfast: Cucumber Melon Smoothie
Morning Snack: Egg Salad Lettuce Cups
Lunch: Rice and Stir-Fried Bok Choy Bowl
Afternoon Snack: Peanut Butter Oat Energy Bites
Dinner: Chicken and Sweet Potato Sheet Pan

Day 19
Breakfast: Papaya Pineapple Smoothie
Morning Snack: Kale Chips
Lunch: Millet and Roasted Eggplant Bowl
Afternoon Snack: Blueberry Chia Pudding
Dinner: Roasted Tofu with Brussels Sprouts

Day 20
Breakfast: Spinach Mango Smoothie
Morning Snack: Peanut Butter and Celery Sticks
Lunch: Buffalo Chicken Wrap
Afternoon Snack: Coconut Almond Energy Balls
Dinner: Shrimp and Lemon Risotto

Day 21
Breakfast: Cinnamon Walnut Overnight Oats
Morning Snack: Gluten-Free Crackers with Avocado Slices
Lunch: Wild Rice and Roasted Bell Pepper Bowl
Afternoon Snack: Almond Butter Rice Cakes
Dinner: Turkey and Bell Pepper Skillet

Day 22
Breakfast: Strawberry Orange Smoothie
Morning Snack: Kale Chips
Lunch: Lentil and Carrot Stew
Afternoon Snack: Peanut Butter Oat Energy Bites
Dinner: Pasta with Roasted Red Pepper Sauce

Day 23
Breakfast: Cottage Cheese and Pineapple Bowl
Morning Snack: Honey Almond Nut Mix
Lunch: Hummus and Cucumber Wrap
Afternoon Snack: Walnut and Date Energy Bites
Dinner: Lemon Herb Tilapia and Broccoli

Day 24
Breakfast: Sweet Potato and Egg Scramble
Morning Snack: Blueberry Almond Granola Bars
Lunch: Quinoa and Roasted Carrot Bowl
Afternoon Snack: Roasted Pumpkin Seeds
Dinner: Roasted Chicken Sausage with Bell Peppers

Maintaining Digestive Health After the 60-Day Plan

Maintaining digestive health after the 60-day Low-FODMAP plan is about taking what you've learned from the elimination and reintroduction phases and incorporating it into your long-term lifestyle. You've worked hard to identify your personal triggers, and now the goal is to maintain a balanced diet that supports your gut health, while still allowing flexibility and variety in your meals. Here's how to navigate this next stage and sustain your digestive well-being beyond the structured phases.

12. Personalized Eating for Long-Term Success

The 60-day plan has shown you which foods trigger symptoms and which ones you can enjoy without issues. Now, it's about fine-tuning your diet to be sustainable over time. This involves making conscious decisions about the types of foods you include in your regular meals, ensuring they align with your tolerance levels while giving you the variety and nutrients your body needs.

At this stage, you're no longer restricted to the rigid structure of the elimination phase, but it's important to remember that balance is key. Some people find they can tolerate small amounts of high-FODMAP foods, while others may need to be more cautious. You're now in a position to decide whether you want to keep certain foods in limited quantities or avoid them altogether.

13. Staying Attuned to Your Body

One of the most important things you've developed over the past 60 days is a heightened awareness of your body's reactions to specific foods. Keep this awareness sharp. It's likely that your tolerance to certain FODMAPs may fluctuate over time due to factors like stress, sleep, and overall health. For instance, during periods of high stress, you might find that even foods you usually tolerate well may start causing mild symptoms. This is normal, and it's a reminder to stay mindful of your body's signals and adjust your diet accordingly.

If you notice new symptoms or patterns, it's worth revisiting your food choices and seeing if there's anything you need to adjust. Your personal triggers may evolve, and that's perfectly fine—as long as you stay flexible and responsive to your body's feedback, you'll be able to maintain digestive health.

14. Balancing Nutrition with Digestive Comfort

While avoiding high-FODMAP foods might feel safe, it's essential to ensure that you're not sacrificing nutrition. Make sure your meals are well-balanced with enough fiber, protein, and healthy fats to support overall health, as well as digestive function. For instance, if you've found that you react to legumes, focus on getting fiber from other sources like low-FODMAP fruits and vegetables, such as carrots, spinach, and berries.

Keep rotating through different low-FODMAP foods to avoid falling into a monotonous routine. A varied diet will help ensure that you're getting a wide range of nutrients, which is essential for maintaining long-term health and energy levels.

15. Strategies for Managing Occasional Flare-Ups

Even with careful planning and awareness, occasional flare-ups can happen. These might occur due to accidental ingestion of trigger foods, stress, or a combination of factors. The key is to know how to manage these flare-ups without letting them derail your progress.

When symptoms arise, return to what you know worked during the elimination phase—stick to low-FODMAP meals that you've identified as "safe" for your gut until your symptoms subside. During flare-ups, hydration and gentle, easy-to-digest meals, such as rice, lean proteins, and cooked vegetables, can help soothe your digestive system.

Additionally, take time to reduce stress levels, as the gut-brain connection plays a significant role in how your digestive system responds to food. Engage in mindfulness, gentle movement, or relaxation techniques to help bring your body back to balance.

16. Social Situations and Travel

One of the ongoing challenges many people face is managing their dietary needs in social situations or while traveling. While you may not always have complete control over your food choices, planning ahead can minimize potential disruptions. For example, when eating out, communicate your needs clearly to restaurant staff, ask for simple modifications to meals, and avoid high-FODMAP triggers that you know may cause symptoms.

When traveling, pack some of your favorite low-FODMAP snacks to ensure you have options on hand if suitable meals aren't available. Keeping your diet stable, even while you're out of your normal routine, is crucial to maintaining digestive health.

17. Long-Term Gut Health Maintenance

As you transition into long-term management of your diet, remember that gut health isn't just about what you eat—it's about your overall lifestyle. Maintaining adequate hydration, regular exercise, and managing stress are all critical factors in keeping your digestive system functioning smoothly.

Probiotics, whether from foods like lactose-free yogurt or from supplements, can also support the health of your gut microbiome. Fiber, as mentioned earlier, remains essential, but make sure you're getting it from low-FODMAP sources that you tolerate well.

18. Flexibility and Reassessing Over Time

Life will inevitably bring changes—whether it's a new work schedule, increased stress, or just getting older—and your digestive needs might shift accordingly. It's okay to revisit your FODMAP triggers every once in a while, especially if you notice changes in how your body reacts to certain foods.

You may find over time that foods that once triggered symptoms become tolerable in moderation. On the other hand, if stress or illness causes more sensitivity, you may need to tighten your diet for a while. The goal is to stay flexible and adjust your eating habits as your body's needs evolve.

PART III: THE LOW-FODMAP RECIPE COLLECTION

In this part of book, we dive into the heart of what makes the Low-FODMAP diet practical and enjoyable—delicious, easy-to-make recipes that nourish your body without triggering symptoms. Whether you're new to the diet or looking for fresh meal ideas, these recipes are designed to make your journey simpler and more fulfilling. Every dish in this section has been carefully crafted with Low-FODMAP ingredients, balancing flavor, nutrition, and ease of preparation. My goal is to give you confidence in the kitchen, so you can enjoy eating while maintaining your digestive health. Let's get cooking!

Chapter 8: Breakfasts on a Budget

Almond Butter Banana Overnight Oats

Preparation Time: 5 minutes
Cooking Time: None
Portions: 1
Ingredients

- ½ cup gluten-free oats
- ½ tablespoon almond butter (unsweetened)
- ½ unripe banana, sliced
- ½ cup lactose-free milk
- 1 teaspoon chia seeds
- 1 teaspoon maple syrup (optional)

Instructions
1. In a jar or bowl, combine the gluten-free oats, almond butter, chia seeds, and lactose-free milk.
2. Add the sliced unripe banana on top and drizzle with maple syrup if desired.
3. Stir gently to combine the ingredients.
4. Cover and refrigerate overnight or for at least 4 hours.
5. Stir before serving and enjoy directly from the jar or transfer to a bowl.

Nutritional Values:
Calories: 260 | Protein: 8g | Fat: 9g | Carbohydrates: 38g | Fiber: 6g | Sugars: 11g

Almond Milk Chia Pudding

Preparation Time: 5 minutes
Cooking Time: None (requires at least 4 hours refrigeration)
Portions: 1
Ingredients

- ½ cup unsweetened almond milk
- 1 tablespoon chia seeds
- ½ teaspoon vanilla extract
- 1 tablespoon maple syrup (optional)
- ¼ cup strawberries, sliced

Instructions
1. In a jar or bowl, combine the gluten-free oats, yogurt, almond milk, chia seeds, and shredded coconut.
2. Add the blueberries on top, then stir gently to mix the ingredients.
3. Cover the jar or bowl and refrigerate overnight or for at least 4 hours.
4. Stir the oats before serving.
5. Enjoy directly from the jar or transfer to a bowl.

Nutritional Values:
Calories: 140 | Protein: 3g | Fat: 7g | Carbohydrates: 17g | Fiber: 6g | Sugars: 7g

Blueberry Coconut Overnight Oats

Preparation Time: 5 minutes
Cooking Time: None
Portions: 1
Ingredients

- ½ cup gluten-free oats
- ½ cup blueberries
- ½ cup lactose-free yogurt
- ½ cup unsweetened almond milk
- 1 tablespoon shredded coconut (unsweetened)
- 1 teaspoon chia seeds

Instructions

1. In a jar or bowl, combine the gluten-free oats, lactose-free yogurt, almond milk, chia seeds, and shredded coconut.
2. Add the blueberries on top and stir gently to combine the ingredients.
3. Cover and refrigerate overnight or for at least 4 hours.
4. Stir before serving and enjoy directly from the jar or transfer to a bowl.

Nutritional Values:
Calories: 280 | Protein: 8g | Fat: 9g | Carbohydrates: 44g | Fiber: 7g | Sugars: 16g

Avocado Kiwi Bowl

Preparation Time: 5 minutes
Cooking Time: None
Portions: 1
Ingredients

- ½ ripe avocado, peeled and chopped
- 1 kiwi, peeled and sliced
- ½ cup lactose-free yogurt
- ½ cup spinach
- 1 tablespoon chia seeds
- 1 tablespoon walnuts (for topping)

Instructions

1. In a blender, combine the avocado, kiwi, lactose-free yogurt, spinach, and chia seeds.
2. Blend until smooth and creamy.
3. Pour the mixture into a bowl.
4. Top with chopped walnuts for added crunch.
5. Enjoy immediately.

Nutritional Values:
Calories: 280 | Protein: 7g | Fat: 20g | Carbohydrates: 20g | Fiber: 9g | Sugars: 10g

Blueberry Spinach Smoothie

Preparation Time: 5 minutes
Cooking Time: None
Portions: 1

Ingredients
- ½ cup blueberries
- ½ cup spinach
- ½ cup lactose-free yogurt
- ½ cup unsweetened almond milk
- ½ cup ice

Instructions
1. Add the blueberries, spinach, lactose-free yogurt, almond milk, and ice to a blender.
2. Blend on high speed until the mixture is smooth and creamy.
3. Pour the smoothie into a glass.
4. Serve immediately and enjoy.

Nutritional Values:
Calories: 140 | Protein: 6g | Fat: 4g | Carbohydrates: 20g | Fiber: 4g | Sugars: 11g

Chive and Cheddar Omelet

Preparation Time: 5 minutes
Cooking Time: 5 minutes
Portions: 1

Ingredients
- 2 large eggs
- 2 tablespoons lactose-free cheddar cheese, shredded
- 1 tablespoon fresh chives, chopped
- 1 teaspoon olive oil
- Salt and pepper to taste

Instructions
1. In a small bowl, whisk the eggs with a pinch of salt and pepper.
2. Heat the olive oil in a non-stick pan over medium heat.
3. Pour the eggs into the pan and let cook for about 2 minutes, until they begin to set.
4. Sprinkle the shredded cheddar and chopped chives over half of the omelet.
5. Fold the omelet in half and cook for another 1-2 minutes, until the cheese is melted, and the eggs are fully cooked.
6. Serve immediately.

Nutritional Values:
Calories: 250 | Protein: 16g | Fat: 20g | Carbohydrates: 2g | Fiber: 0g | Sugars: 1g

Cinnamon Walnut Overnight Oats

Preparation Time: 5 minutes
Cooking Time: None
Portions: 1
Ingredients
- ½ cup gluten-free oats
- ½ cup lactose-free almond milk
- 1 tablespoon chopped walnuts
- 1 teaspoon ground cinnamon
- 1 teaspoon chia seeds
- 1 teaspoon maple syrup (optional)

Instructions
1. In a jar or bowl, combine the gluten-free oats, almond milk, cinnamon, chia seeds, and maple syrup if using.
2. Stir in the chopped walnuts.
3. Cover and refrigerate overnight or for at least 4 hours.
4. Stir before serving and enjoy directly from the jar or transfer to a bowl.

Nutritional Values:
Calories: 270 | Protein: 6g | Fat: 11g | Carbohydrates: 37g | Fiber: 6g | Sugars: 8g

Cottage Cheese and Pineapple Bowl

Preparation Time: 5 minutes
Cooking Time: None
Portions: 1
Ingredients
- ½ cup lactose-free cottage cheese
- ½ cup pineapple chunks
- 1 tablespoon walnuts, chopped
- 1 teaspoon chia seeds

Instructions
1. Scoop the lactose-free cottage cheese into a serving bowl.
2. Evenly top the cottage cheese with the pineapple chunks.
3. Sprinkle the chopped walnuts over the pineapple.
4. Add a final sprinkle of chia seeds for texture.
5. Serve immediately and enjoy.

Nutritional Values:
Calories: 180 | Protein: 10g | Fat: 7g | Carbohydrates: 19g | Fiber: 2g | Sugars: 13g

Cucumber Kiwi Bowl

Preparation Time: 5 minutes
Cooking Time: None
Portions: 1
Ingredients
- ½ cup cucumber, peeled and chopped
- 1 kiwi, peeled and sliced
- ½ cup lactose-free yogurt
- ½ cup spinach
- 1 tablespoon chia seeds
- 1 tablespoon walnuts (for topping)

Instructions
1. In a blender, combine the cucumber, kiwi, lactose-free yogurt, spinach, and chia seeds.
2. Blend until smooth and creamy.
3. Pour the mixture into a bowl.
4. Top with chopped walnuts for added texture.
5. Enjoy immediately.

Nutritional Values:
Calories: 190 | Protein: 6g | Fat: 10g | Carbohydrates: 22g | Fiber: 6g | Sugars: 12g

Cucumber Melon Smoothie

Preparation Time: 5 minutes
Cooking Time: None
Portions: 1
Ingredients:
- ½ cup cucumber, peeled and chopped
- ½ cup cantaloupe, cubed
- ½ cup lactose-free yogurt
- 4-5 fresh mint leaves
- ½ cup water
- ½ cup ice

Instructions:
1. In a blender, combine the cucumber, cantaloupe, lactose-free yogurt, fresh mint leaves, and water.
2. Add ice cubes to the blender.
3. Blend on high until the mixture is smooth and creamy.
4. Pour into a glass and enjoy immediately.

Nutritional Values:
Calories: 120 | Protein: 5g | Fat: 2g | Carbohydrates: 20g | Fiber: 2g | Sugars: 15g

Egg and Avocado Breakfast Wrap

Preparation Time: 5 minutes
Cooking Time: 5 minutes
Portions: 1
Ingredients
- 2 large eggs, scrambled
- ¼ avocado, sliced
- 1 gluten-free tortilla
- ¼ cup spinach
- 1 teaspoon olive oil

Instructions
1. Heat the olive oil in a pan over medium heat, then scramble the eggs until fully cooked.
2. Warm the gluten-free tortilla slightly if desired.
3. Place the scrambled eggs onto the center of the tortilla.
4. Add the avocado slices and spinach on top of the eggs.
5. Fold the tortilla into a wrap and serve immediately.

Nutritional Values:
Calories: 270 | Protein: 12g | Fat: 18g | Carbohydrates: 18g | Fiber: 4g | Sugars: 1g

Gluten-Free Toast with Peanut Butter and Blueberries

Preparation Time: 5 minutes
Cooking Time: 2 minutes
Portions: 1
Ingredients
- 1 slice gluten-free bread
- 1 tablespoon peanut butter (unsweetened)
- ¼ cup blueberries
- 1 teaspoon chia seeds

Instructions
1. Toast the gluten-free bread.
2. Spread peanut butter on the toast.
3. Top with blueberries and chia seeds.

Nutritional Values:
Calories: 220 | Protein: 7g | Fat: 10g | Carbohydrates: 28g | Fiber: 5g | Sugars: 7g

Kiwi Pineapple Smoothie

Preparation Time: 5 minutes
Cooking Time: None
Portions: 1
Ingredients
- 1 kiwi, peeled and chopped
- ½ cup pineapple, cubed
- ½ cup lactose-free milk
- ½ cup spinach
- 1 tablespoon chia seeds
- ½ cup ice

Instructions
1. Place the kiwi, pineapple, lactose-free milk, spinach, and chia seeds into a blender.
2. Add ice cubes to the blender.
3. Blend until smooth and creamy.
4. Pour into a glass and serve immediately.

Nutritional Values:
Calories: 160 | Protein: 5g | Fat: 4g | Carbohydrates: 30g | Fiber: 5g | Sugars: 18g

Oatmeal with Almonds and Maple Syrup

Preparation Time: 5 minutes
Cooking Time: 5 minutes
Portions: 1
Ingredients
- ½ cup gluten-free oats
- 1 cup unsweetened almond milk
- 1 tablespoon sliced almonds
- 1 teaspoon maple syrup

Instructions
1. In a small pot, combine the gluten-free oats and almond milk.
2. Cook the mixture over medium heat, stirring occasionally, until the oats thicken, about 5 minutes.
3. Once thickened, remove the pot from heat and stir in the maple syrup.
4. Transfer the oatmeal to a serving bowl.
5. Top with sliced almonds and serve immediately.

Nutritional Values:
Calories: 200 | Protein: 5g | Fat: 7g | Carbohydrates: 32g | Fiber: 5g | Sugars: 8g

Papaya Pineapple Smoothie

Preparation Time: 5 minutes
Cooking Time: None
Portions: 1
Ingredients
- ½ cup papaya, peeled and cubed
- ½ cup pineapple, cubed
- ½ cup lactose-free yogurt
- ½ cup unsweetened almond milk
- 1 tablespoon flaxseeds
- ½ cup ice

Instructions
1. In a blender, combine the papaya, pineapple, lactose-free yogurt, almond milk, and flaxseeds.
2. Add ice cubes and blend until smooth and creamy.
3. Pour into a glass and enjoy immediately.

Nutritional Values:
Calories: 190 | Protein: 5g | Fat: 5g | Carbohydrates: 33g | Fiber: 5g | Sugars: 23g

Peanut Butter Banana Smoothie

Preparation Time: 5 minutes
Cooking Time: None
Portions: 1
Ingredients
- 1 unripe banana, peeled and sliced
- 1 tablespoon natural peanut butter (no added sweeteners)
- ½ cup unsweetened almond milk
- ½ cup spinach
- 1 tablespoon flaxseeds
- ½ cup ice

Instructions
1. Add the banana, peanut butter, almond milk, spinach, and flaxseeds to a blender.
2. Add ice cubes and blend until smooth and creamy.
3. Pour into a glass and enjoy immediately.

Nutritional Values:
Calories: 210 | Protein: 6g | Fat: 10g | Carbohydrates: 28g | Fiber: 6g | Sugars: 10g

Pineapple Ginger Smoothie

Preparation Time: 5 minutes
Cooking Time: None
Portions: 1
Ingredients
- ½ cup pineapple, cubed
- ½ teaspoon fresh ginger, grated
- ½ cup lactose-free yogurt
- ½ cup unsweetened almond milk
- 1 tablespoon chia seeds
- ½ cup ice

Instructions
1. In a blender, combine the pineapple, grated ginger, lactose-free yogurt, almond milk, and chia seeds.
2. Add ice cubes and blend until smooth and creamy.
3. Pour into a glass and enjoy immediately.

Nutritional Values:
Calories: 160 | Protein: 5g | Fat: 4g | Carbohydrates: 28g | Fiber: 4g | Sugars: 20g

Rice Cakes with Smoked Salmon and Cucumbers

Preparation Time: 5 minutes
Cooking Time: None
Portions: 1
Ingredients
- 2 rice cakes
- 2 slices smoked salmon
- ¼ cucumber, thinly sliced
- 1 tablespoon lactose-free cream cheese
- 1 teaspoon fresh dill (optional)

Instructions
1. Spread the lactose-free cream cheese evenly over both rice cakes.
2. Place a slice of smoked salmon on top of each cream cheese-covered rice cake.
3. Arrange thinly sliced cucumber over the smoked salmon.
4. If desired, sprinkle fresh dill on top for extra flavor.
5. Serve immediately and enjoy.

Nutritional Values:
Calories: 180 | Protein: 10g | Fat: 6g | Carbohydrates: 20g | Fiber: 1g | Sugars: 2g

Scrambled Eggs with Bell Peppers

Preparation Time: 5 minutes
Cooking Time: 5 minutes
Portions: 1
Ingredients
- 2 large eggs
- ¼ cup red bell pepper, diced
- ¼ cup green bell pepper, diced
- 1 teaspoon olive oil
- Salt and pepper to taste

Instructions
1. In a small bowl, whisk the eggs with a pinch of salt and pepper.
2. Heat olive oil in a non-stick pan over medium heat.
3. Add the diced red and green bell peppers to the pan and sauté for 2-3 minutes, until softened.
4. Pour in the whisked eggs and cook, stirring gently, until scrambled and fully set.
5. Serve immediately and enjoy.

Nutritional Values:
Calories: 180 | Protein: 12g | Fat: 14g | Carbohydrates: 4g | Fiber: 1g | Sugars: 2g

Smoothie Bowl with Mango and Spinach

Preparation Time: 5 minutes
Cooking Time: None
Portions: 1
Ingredients
- ½ cup mango, cubed
- ½ cup spinach
- ½ cup lactose-free yogurt
- ½ cup almond milk
- 1 tablespoon chia seeds

Instructions
1. Blend the mango, spinach, yogurt, and almond milk until smooth.
2. Pour into a bowl and top with chia seeds.
3. Serve immediately.

Nutritional Values:
Calories: 190 | Protein: 7g | Fat: 4g | Carbohydrates: 34g | Fiber: 6g | Sugars: 20g

Spinach and Blueberry Smoothie Bowl

Preparation Time: 5 minutes
Cooking Time: None
Portions: 1
Ingredients
- ½ cup fresh spinach
- ½ cup blueberries
- ½ cup lactose-free yogurt
- ½ cup unsweetened almond milk
- 1 tablespoon chia seeds
- 2 tablespoons gluten-free oats (for topping)

Instructions
1. In a blender, combine the spinach, blueberries, lactose-free yogurt, almond milk, and chia seeds.
2. Blend until smooth and creamy.
3. Pour the smoothie into a bowl.
4. Top with gluten-free oats for added texture.
5. Enjoy immediately.

Nutritional Values:
Calories: 180 | Protein: 6g | Fat: 5g | Carbohydrates: 30g | Fiber: 7g | Sugars: 15g

Spinach Mango Smoothie

Preparation Time: 5 minutes
Cooking Time: None
Portions: 1
Ingredients
- ½ cup mango, cubed
- ½ cup fresh spinach
- ½ cup lactose-free milk
- 1 tablespoon chia seeds
- ½ cup ice

Instructions
1. In a blender, combine the mango, spinach, lactose-free milk, and chia seeds.
2. Add ice cubes and blend until smooth and creamy.
3. Pour into a glass and enjoy immediately.

Nutritional Values:
Calories: 150 | Protein: 5g | Fat: 3g | Carbohydrates: 28g | Fiber: 5g | Sugars: 20g

Strawberry Almond Overnight Oats

Preparation Time: 5 minutes
Cooking Time: None
Portions: 1
Ingredients
- ½ cup gluten-free oats
- ½ cup strawberries, sliced
- ½ cup unsweetened almond milk
- 1 tablespoon almond butter (unsweetened)
- 1 teaspoon chia seeds
- ½ teaspoon vanilla extract (optional)

Instructions
1. In a jar or bowl, combine the gluten-free oats, almond milk, almond butter, chia seeds, and vanilla extract (if using).
2. Stir in the sliced strawberries.
3. Mix well to ensure all ingredients are combined.
4. Cover and refrigerate overnight or for at least 4 hours.
5. Stir before serving and enjoy directly from the jar or transfer to a bowl.

Nutritional Values (per serving):
Calories: 280 | Protein: 8g | Fat: 12g | Carbohydrates: 37g | Fiber: 8g | Sugars: 9g

Strawberry Orange Smoothie

Preparation Time: 5 minutes
Cooking Time: None
Portions: 1
Ingredients
- ½ cup strawberries, hulled
- 1 small orange, peeled and segmented
- ½ cup lactose-free yogurt
- ½ cup almond milk
- 1 tablespoon flaxseeds
- ½ cup ice

Instructions
1. Combine the strawberries, orange segments, lactose-free yogurt, almond milk, and flaxseeds in a blender.
2. Add ice cubes to the mixture.
3. Blend on high until smooth and creamy.
4. Pour into a glass and enjoy immediately.

Nutritional Values:
Calories: 170 | Protein: 5g | Fat: 6g | Carbohydrates: 28g | Fiber: 5g | Sugars: 20g

Sweet Potato and Egg Scramble

Preparation Time: 5 minutes
Cooking Time: 10 minutes
Portions: 1
Ingredients
- ½ cup sweet potato, peeled and cubed (pre-cooked or steamed)
- 2 large eggs
- 1 tablespoon olive oil
- ¼ cup fresh spinach, chopped
- Salt and pepper to taste

Instructions
1. Heat the olive oil in a non-stick pan over medium heat.
2. Add the pre-cooked sweet potato cubes to the pan and cook for 2-3 minutes, stirring occasionally, until slightly crispy.
3. Stir in the chopped spinach and cook for another 1-2 minutes, until wilted.
4. In a small bowl, whisk the eggs with a pinch of salt and pepper.
5. Pour the eggs into the pan and scramble gently until fully cooked and combined with the sweet potato and spinach.
6. Serve immediately and enjoy.

Nutritional Values:
Calories: 260 | Protein: 10g | Fat: 16g | Carbohydrates: 19g | Fiber: 3g | Sugars: 4g

Chapter 9 (25 recipes): Fast and Easy Lunches

Avocado and Egg Salad Sandwich

Preparation Time: 10 minutes
Cooking Time: None
Portions: 1
Ingredients

- 2 hard-boiled eggs, chopped
- ½ avocado, mashed
- 1 tablespoon lactose-free mayonnaise
- 2 slices gluten-free bread
- Lettuce

Instructions
1. In a bowl, combine the chopped eggs, mashed avocado, and mayonnaise.
2. Spread the mixture on one slice of gluten-free bread.
3. Add lettuce and top with the other slice of bread.
4. Cut in half and serve.

Nutritional Values:
Calories: 340 | Protein: 14g | Fat: 24g | Carbohydrates: 22g | Fiber: 6g | Sugars: 2g

Avocado and Tuna Salad

Preparation Time: 5 minutes
Cooking Time: None
Portions: 1
Ingredients

- 1 can tuna (drained)
- ½ avocado, diced
- 1 cup spinach
- 1 tablespoon olive oil
- 1 teaspoon lemon juice
- Salt to taste

Instructions
1. In a bowl, combine the drained tuna and diced avocado.
2. Add the spinach to the bowl with the tuna and avocado.
3. Drizzle with olive oil and lemon juice.
4. Season with salt to taste and mix gently.
5. Serve immediately and enjoy.

Nutritional Values:
Calories: 320 | Protein: 24g | Fat: 22g | Carbohydrates: 6g | Fiber: 5g | Sugars: 1g

Brown Rice and Kale Bowl

Preparation Time: 10 minutes
Cooking Time: 15 minutes
Portions: 1
Ingredients
- ½ cup cooked brown rice
- ½ cup sautéed kale
- ½ cup grilled salmon, sliced
- 1 tablespoon olive oil
- 1 teaspoon lemon juice

Instructions
1. Heat the olive oil in a pan and sauté the kale for 3-4 minutes until tender.
2. In a serving bowl, layer the cooked brown rice at the bottom.
3. Add the sautéed kale on top of the rice.
4. Place the grilled salmon slices on top of the kale.
5. Drizzle with lemon juice and serve warm.

Nutritional Values:
Calories: 400 | Protein: 24g | Fat: 18g | Carbohydrates: 36g | Fiber: 5g | Sugars: 2g

Brown Rice and Roasted Carrot Bowl

Preparation Time: 10 minutes
Cooking Time: 30 minutes
Portions: 1
Ingredients
- ½ cup cooked brown rice
- ½ cup roasted carrots
- 1 cup spinach
- 1 tablespoon olive oil
- 1 teaspoon lemon juice
- ½ cup grilled chicken, sliced

Instructions
1. Preheat the oven to 400°F (200°C) and roast the carrots for 25-30 minutes until tender.
2. In a serving bowl, layer the cooked brown rice and fresh spinach.
3. Add the roasted carrots and sliced grilled chicken on top of the rice and spinach.
4. Drizzle with olive oil and lemon juice for added flavor.
5. Serve warm and enjoy.

Nutritional Values:
Calories: 380 | Protein: 24g | Fat: 14g | Carbohydrates: 42g | Fiber: 6g | Sugars: 5g

Buckwheat and Zucchini Bowl

Preparation Time: 10 minutes
Cooking Time: 20 minutes
Portions: 1
Ingredients
- ½ cup cooked buckwheat
- ½ cup sautéed zucchini
- 2 tablespoons lactose-free feta
- 1 tablespoon olive oil
- ½ cup grilled shrimp

Instructions
1. Sauté the zucchini in olive oil for 5-7 minutes until tender.
2. In a bowl, layer the cooked buckwheat and zucchini.
3. Top with grilled shrimp and crumbled feta.
4. Serve warm.

Nutritional Values:

Calories: 360 | Protein: 22g | Fat: 16g | Carbohydrates: 32g | Fiber: 5g | Sugars: 3g

Buffalo Chicken Wrap

Preparation Time: 10 minutes
Cooking Time: 10 minutes (for cooking chicken)
Portions: 1
Ingredients
- ½ cup grilled chicken, chopped
- 1 tablespoon lactose-free ranch dressing
- 1 tablespoon buffalo sauce (low-FODMAP)
- 1 gluten-free tortilla
- Lettuce
- Shredded carrots

Instructions
1. Mix the grilled chicken with buffalo sauce.
2. Layer the tortilla with lettuce, shredded carrots, and chicken.
3. Drizzle with ranch dressing.
4. Wrap tightly and serve.

Nutritional Values:

Calories: 290 | Protein: 23g | Fat: 12g | Carbohydrates: 25g | Fiber: 3g | Sugars: 2g

Caprese Wrap

Preparation Time: 5 minutes
Cooking Time: None
Portions: 1
Ingredients
- ¼ cup lactose-free mozzarella, sliced
- ¼ cup cherry tomatoes, halved
- Fresh basil leaves
- 1 gluten-free tortilla
- 1 tablespoon olive oil
- 1 teaspoon balsamic vinegar

Instructions
1. Layer the tortilla with mozzarella slices, cherry tomatoes, and basil leaves.
2. Drizzle with olive oil and balsamic vinegar.
3. Wrap tightly and serve.

Nutritional Values:
Calories: 240 | Protein: 10g | Fat: 16g | Carbohydrates: 15g | Fiber: 2g | Sugars: 3g

Chicken and Rice Stir-Fry

Preparation Time: 5 minutes
Cooking Time: 10 minutes
Portions: 1
Ingredients
- ½ cup cooked chicken, shredded
- ½ cup cooked brown rice
- ¼ cup shredded carrots
- 1 cup spinach
- 1 tablespoon olive oil
- 1 tablespoon gluten-free soy sauce

Instructions
1. Heat olive oil in a pan over medium heat.
2. Add shredded carrots and cook for 2-3 minutes.
3. Stir in cooked chicken, rice, and spinach, and cook for another 2-3 minutes.
4. Add gluten-free soy sauce and stir well.
5. Serve immediately.

Nutritional Values:
Calories: 350 | Protein: 24g | Fat: 12g | Carbohydrates: 38g | Fiber: 4g | Sugars: 2g

Coconut Shrimp and Rice

Preparation Time: 10 minutes
Cooking Time: 10 minutes
Portions: 1
Ingredients
- ½ cup shrimp, peeled and deveined
- ½ cup white rice (cooked)
- ¼ cup coconut milk (low-FODMAP)
- 1 cup spinach
- 1 tablespoon olive oil
- 1 teaspoon lime juice

Instructions
1. Heat olive oil in a skillet over medium heat.
2. Add shrimp and cook for 2-3 minutes until pink.
3. Add spinach and cook until wilted, about 2 minutes.
4. Stir in coconut milk and lime juice and cook for another 2 minutes.
5. Serve over the cooked white rice.

Nutritional Values:
Calories: 350 | Protein: 22g | Fat: 16g | Carbohydrates: 30g | Fiber: 3g | Sugars: 2g

Egg and Potato Salad

Preparation Time: 10 minutes
Cooking Time: 15 minutes
Portions: 1
Ingredients
- 2 hard-boiled eggs, chopped
- ½ cup boiled potatoes, diced
- 1 tablespoon lactose-free mayonnaise
- 1 cup spinach
- 1 tablespoon olive oil
- 1 teaspoon mustard

Instructions
1. In a bowl, combine the chopped hard-boiled eggs, diced boiled potatoes, mayonnaise, and mustard.
2. Add the spinach to the mixture.
3. Drizzle with olive oil and gently toss all the ingredients together.
4. Mix until evenly combined.
5. Serve immediately and enjoy.

Nutritional Values:
Calories: 320 | Protein: 12g | Fat: 22g | Carbohydrates: 22g | Fiber: 3g | Sugars: 1g

Ground Turkey and Sweet Potato Skillet

Preparation Time: 10 minutes
Cooking Time: 20 minutes
Portions: 1
Ingredients
- ½ cup ground turkey
- ½ cup diced sweet potatoes
- 1 cup spinach
- 1 tablespoon olive oil
- ½ teaspoon cumin
- Salt to taste

Instructions
1. Heat olive oil in a skillet over medium heat.
2. Add diced sweet potatoes and cook for 8-10 minutes until tender.
3. Stir in ground turkey and cook until browned, about 5-7 minutes.
4. Add spinach, cumin, and salt, cooking until the spinach wilts.
5. Serve warm.

Nutritional Values:
Calories: 340 | Protein: 24g | Fat: 16g | Carbohydrates: 30g | Fiber: 4g | Sugars: 4g

Ham and Spinach Sandwich

Preparation Time: 5 minutes
Cooking Time: None
Portions: 1
Ingredients
- 2 slices gluten-free bread
- 2 slices ham (low-FODMAP)
- 1 slice lactose-free Swiss cheese
- 1 handful spinach
- Mustard

Instructions
1. Spread mustard on one slice of bread.
2. Layer with ham, Swiss cheese, and spinach.
3. Top with the second slice of bread.
4. Serve immediately.

Nutritional Values:
Calories: 280 | Protein: 18g | Fat: 12g | Carbohydrates: 28g | Fiber: 4g | Sugars: 2g

Hummus and Cucumber Wrap

Preparation Time: 5 minutes
Cooking Time: None
Portions: 1
Ingredients
- 1 gluten-free tortilla
- 2 tablespoons low-FODMAP hummus
- ½ cucumber, sliced
- 1 cup spinach
- 1 teaspoon olive oil

Instructions
1. Spread hummus on the tortilla.
2. Layer with cucumber slices and spinach.
3. Drizzle with olive oil, wrap tightly, and serve.

Nutritional Values:
Calories: 240 | Protein: 7g | Fat: 12g | Carbohydrates: 28g | Fiber: 6g | Sugars: 3g

Lentil and Carrot Stew

Preparation Time: 5 minutes
Cooking Time: 20 minutes
Portions: 1
Ingredients
- ½ cup lentils
- ½ cup diced carrots
- 1 cup spinach
- 1 tablespoon olive oil
- 1 cup gluten-free vegetable broth
- Salt to taste

Instructions
1. In a pot, heat olive oil and sauté carrots for 3-4 minutes.
2. Add lentils and vegetable broth and bring to a boil.
3. Reduce heat and simmer for 15-20 minutes until lentils are tender.
4. Stir in spinach and cook for an additional 2 minutes.
5. Season with salt and serve.

Nutritional Values:
Calories: 290 | Protein: 14g | Fat: 8g | Carbohydrates: 42g | Fiber: 10g | Sugars: 5g

Millet and Grilled Zucchini Bowl

Preparation Time: 10 minutes
Cooking Time: 15 minutes
Portions: 1
Ingredients
- ½ cup cooked millet
- ½ cup grilled zucchini
- 2 tablespoons lactose-free feta
- 1 cup spinach
- 1 tablespoon olive oil

Instructions
1. Grill the zucchini for 3-4 minutes per side until tender.
2. In a bowl, layer the cooked millet and spinach.
3. Add the grilled zucchini and crumbled feta.
4. Drizzle with olive oil and serve warm.

Nutritional Values:

Calories: 320 | Protein: 10g | Fat: 14g | Carbohydrates: 40g | Fiber: 6g | Sugars: 3g

Millet and Roasted Eggplant Bowl

Preparation Time: 10 minutes
Cooking Time: 25 minutes
Portions: 1
Ingredients
- ½ cup cooked millet
- ½ cup roasted eggplant
- 1 cup spinach
- 2 tablespoons lactose-free feta
- 1 tablespoon olive oil

Instructions
1. Preheat the oven to 400°F (200°C) and roast the eggplant for 20-25 minutes until tender.
2. In a serving bowl, layer the cooked millet and fresh spinach.
3. Add the roasted eggplant on top of the millet and spinach.
4. Crumble the lactose-free feta over the roasted eggplant.
5. Drizzle with olive oil and serve warm.

Nutritional Values:

Calories: 340 | Protein: 10g | Fat: 15g | Carbohydrates: 42g | Fiber: 7g | Sugars: 5g

Quinoa and Roasted Vegetable Salad

Preparation Time: 10 minutes
Cooking Time: 25 minutes
Portions: 1
Ingredients
- ½ cup cooked quinoa
- ½ cup roasted carrots
- 1 cup spinach
- 1 tablespoon olive oil
- 1 teaspoon lemon juice

Instructions
1. Preheat oven to 400°F (200°C) and roast carrots for 20-25 minutes until tender.
2. In a bowl, combine cooked quinoa, roasted carrots, and spinach.
3. Drizzle with olive oil and lemon juice.
4. Toss and serve.

Nutritional Values:
Calories: 270 | Protein: 8g | Fat: 14g | Carbohydrates: 30g | Fiber: 6g | Sugars: 5g

Quinoa and Sweet Potato Bowl

Preparation Time: 10 minutes
Cooking Time: 25 minutes
Portions: 1
Ingredients
- ½ cup cooked quinoa
- ½ cup roasted sweet potatoes
- 1 cup spinach
- 1 tablespoon olive oil
- ½ cup grilled chicken, sliced

Instructions
1. Preheat the oven to 400°F (200°C) and roast the sweet potatoes for 20-25 minutes until tender.
2. In a serving bowl, layer the cooked quinoa and fresh spinach.
3. Add the roasted sweet potatoes and sliced grilled chicken on top.
4. Drizzle with olive oil for added flavor.
5. Serve warm and enjoy.

Nutritional Values:
Calories: 370 | Protein: 24g | Fat: 14g | Carbohydrates: 40g | Fiber: 6g | Sugars: 6g

Quinoa and Roasted Bell Pepper Bowl

Preparation Time: 10 minutes
Cooking Time: 25 minutes
Portions: 1
Ingredients
- ½ cup cooked quinoa
- ½ cup roasted bell peppers
- 2 tablespoons lactose-free cheddar cheese, shredded
- 1 cup spinach
- 1 tablespoon olive oil

Instructions
1. Preheat the oven to 400°F (200°C) and roast the bell peppers for 20-25 minutes.
2. In a bowl, layer the cooked quinoa and spinach.
3. Add the roasted bell peppers and shredded cheddar cheese.
4. Drizzle with olive oil and serve warm.

Nutritional Values:
Calories: 330 | Protein: 12g | Fat: 16g | Carbohydrates: 36g | Fiber: 6g | Sugars: 5g

Quinoa and Roasted Carrot Bowl

Preparation Time: 10 minutes
Cooking Time: 25 minutes
Portions: 1
Ingredients
- ½ cup cooked quinoa
- ½ cup roasted carrots
- 1 cup spinach
- 1 tablespoon olive oil
- 1 teaspoon lemon juice

Instructions
1. Preheat the oven to 400°F (200°C) and roast the carrots for 20-25 minutes until tender.
2. In a serving bowl, layer the cooked quinoa and fresh spinach.
3. Add the roasted carrots on top of the quinoa and spinach.
4. Drizzle with olive oil and lemon juice for extra flavor.
5. Serve warm and enjoy.

Nutritional Values:
Calories: 300 | Protein: 8g | Fat: 14g | Carbohydrates: 36g | Fiber: 6g | Sugars: 5g

Rice and Stir-Fried Bok Choy Bowl

Preparation Time: 10 minutes
Cooking Time: 15 minutes
Portions: 1
Ingredients
- ½ cup cooked white rice
- ½ cup stir-fried bok choy
- ½ cup grilled tofu
- 1 teaspoon sesame oil
- 1 cup spinach

Instructions
1. Heat sesame oil in a pan and stir-fry the bok choy for 3-4 minutes until tender.
2. In a serving bowl, layer the cooked white rice and fresh spinach.
3. Add the stir-fried bok choy and grilled tofu on top of the rice and spinach.
4. Serve warm and enjoy.

Nutritional Values:
Calories: 320 | Protein: 14g | Fat: 10g | Carbohydrates: 40g | Fiber: 5g | Sugars: 3g

Rice and Turkey Lettuce Wraps

Preparation Time: 5 minutes
Cooking Time: None
Portions: 1
Ingredients
- ½ cup cooked white rice
- 2 slices turkey breast
- 2 large lettuce leaves
- 1 teaspoon olive oil
- 1 teaspoon mustard

Instructions
1. Lay out the lettuce leaves and place turkey slices and rice in each leaf.
2. Drizzle with olive oil and mustard.
3. Roll the lettuce leaves like wraps and serve.

Nutritional Values:
Calories: 220 | Protein: 14g | Fat: 8g | Carbohydrates: 24g | Fiber: 2g | Sugars: 1g

Spinach and Feta Scramble

Preparation Time: 5 minutes
Cooking Time: 5 minutes
Portions: 1
Ingredients
- 2 large eggs
- ¼ cup lactose-free feta cheese
- 1 cup spinach
- 1 tablespoon olive oil
- Salt and pepper to taste

Instructions
1. Heat olive oil in a pan over medium heat.
2. Add spinach and sauté for 1-2 minutes until wilted.
3. Crack the eggs into the pan and scramble with spinach.
4. Add feta cheese and cook until eggs are fully set.
5. Season with salt and pepper and serve.

Nutritional Values:
Calories: 260 | Protein: 16g | Fat: 20g | Carbohydrates: 4g | Fiber: 2g | Sugars: 1g

Sweet Potato and Black Bean Bowl

Preparation Time: 10 minutes
Cooking Time: 25 minutes
Portions: 1
Ingredients
- ½ cup roasted sweet potatoes
- ½ cup canned black beans (rinsed)
- 1 cup spinach
- 1 tablespoon olive oil
- ¼ teaspoon cumin

Instructions
1. Preheat the oven to 400°F (200°C) and roast the sweet potatoes for 20-25 minutes until tender.
2. In a serving bowl, combine the roasted sweet potatoes, rinsed black beans, and fresh spinach.
3. Drizzle with olive oil and sprinkle with cumin for added flavor.
4. Toss everything together to mix well.
5. Serve warm and enjoy.

Nutritional Values:
Calories: 300 | Protein: 10g | Fat: 12g | Carbohydrates: 40g | Fiber: 10g | Sugars: 7g

Wild Rice and Roasted Bell Pepper Bowl

Preparation Time: 10 minutes
Cooking Time: 25 minutes
Portions: 1
Ingredients
- ½ cup cooked wild rice
- ½ cup roasted bell peppers
- ½ cup grilled chicken, sliced
- 1 cup spinach
- 1 tablespoon olive oil

Instructions
1. Preheat the oven to 400°F (200°C) and roast the bell peppers for 20-25 minutes.
2. In a bowl, layer the cooked wild rice and spinach.
3. Add the roasted bell peppers and grilled chicken.
4. Drizzle with olive oil and serve warm.

Nutritional Values:
Calories: 370 | Protein: 22g | Fat: 14g | Carbohydrates: 38g | Fiber: 6g | Sugars: 4g

Chapter 10 (25 recipes): Effortless Dinners

Baked Lemon Chicken and Green Beans

Preparation Time: 10 minutes
Cooking Time: 25 minutes
Portions: 1
Ingredients

- 1 chicken breast
- 1 cup green beans
- 1 tablespoon olive oil
- 2 lemon slices
- ½ teaspoon thyme
- Salt and pepper to taste

Instructions
1. Preheat the oven to 400°F (200°C).
2. Place the chicken breast and green beans on a sheet pan.
3. Drizzle with olive oil, sprinkle with thyme, salt, and pepper.
4. Top the chicken with lemon slices.
5. Bake for 25 minutes or until the chicken is fully cooked.
6. Serve warm.

Nutritional Values:

Calories: 320 | Protein: 30g | Fat: 15g | Carbohydrates: 12g | Fiber: 4g | Sugars: 2g

Balsamic Glazed Salmon and Asparagus

Preparation Time: 10 minutes
Cooking Time: 20 minutes
Portions: 1
Ingredients

- 1 salmon fillet
- 1 cup asparagus
- 1 tablespoon balsamic vinegar
- 1 tablespoon olive oil
- 1 tablespoon garlic-infused oil
- Salt and pepper to taste

Instructions
1. Preheat the oven to 400°F (200°C).
2. Place the salmon fillet and asparagus on a sheet pan.
3. Drizzle with olive oil and balsamic vinegar.
4. Add garlic-infused oil, salt, and pepper.
5. Bake for 20 minutes or until the salmon is fully cooked.
6. Serve warm.

Nutritional Values:

Calories: 350 | Protein: 28g | Fat: 22g | Carbohydrates: 7g | Fiber: 3g | Sugars: 3g

Basil Pesto Quinoa

Preparation Time: 10 minutes
Cooking Time: 15 minutes
Portions: 1
Ingredients

- ½ cup cooked quinoa
- 1 cup spinach
- 2 tablespoons lactose-free Parmesan cheese
- 1 tablespoon olive oil
- ¼ cup fresh basil
- 1 tablespoon pine nuts

Instructions

1. In a food processor, blend the fresh basil, pine nuts, olive oil, and lactose-free Parmesan until smooth to create the pesto.
2. In a serving bowl, combine the cooked quinoa and fresh spinach.
3. Add the freshly made pesto to the quinoa and spinach, mixing well.
4. Toss until evenly coated with the pesto.
5. Serve warm and enjoy.

Nutritional Values:
Calories: 340 | Protein: 10g | Fat: 18g | Carbohydrates: 32g | Fiber: 5g | Sugars: 2g

Beef and Bell Pepper Fajitas

Preparation Time: 10 minutes
Cooking Time: 15 minutes
Portions: 1
Ingredients

- ½ cup sliced beef
- 1 bell pepper, sliced
- 1 tablespoon olive oil
- 1 teaspoon cumin
- 1 teaspoon lime juice
- Salt to taste

Instructions

1. Preheat the oven to 400°F (200°C).
2. Place the beef and bell peppers on a sheet pan.
3. Drizzle with olive oil, sprinkle with cumin, and squeeze lime juice over.
4. Add salt and toss to coat.
5. Bake for 15 minutes or until the beef is cooked through.
6. Serve warm.

Nutritional Values:
Calories: 300 | Protein: 22g | Fat: 18g | Carbohydrates: 10g | Fiber: 3g | Sugars: 5g

Beef and Quinoa Skillet

Preparation Time: 10 minutes
Cooking Time: 15 minutes
Portions: 1
Ingredients
- ½ cup ground beef
- ½ cup cooked quinoa
- 1 cup spinach
- ¼ cup shredded carrots
- 1 tablespoon olive oil
- 1 tablespoon gluten-free soy sauce

Instructions
1. Heat olive oil in a skillet over medium heat.
2. Add ground beef and cook until browned, about 5-7 minutes.
3. Stir in shredded carrots and cook for another 2 minutes.
4. Add the cooked quinoa, spinach, and soy sauce. Stir well and cook until the spinach wilts.
5. Serve warm.

Nutritional Values:
Calories: 380 | Protein: 24g | Fat: 20g | Carbohydrates: 28g | Fiber: 5g | Sugars: 2g

Chicken and Sweet Potato Sheet Pan

Preparation Time: 10 minutes
Cooking Time: 25 minutes
Portions: 1
Ingredients
- 1 chicken thigh
- ½ cup sweet potatoes, diced
- 1 tablespoon olive oil
- 1 teaspoon rosemary
- Salt and pepper to taste

Instructions
1. Preheat the oven to 400°F (200°C).
2. Place the chicken thigh and diced sweet potatoes on a sheet pan.
3. Drizzle with olive oil, sprinkle with rosemary, salt, and pepper.
4. Bake for 25 minutes or until the chicken is fully cooked and sweet potatoes are tender.
5. Serve warm.

Nutritional Values:
Calories: 350 | Protein: 24g | Fat: 18g | Carbohydrates: 22g | Fiber: 4g | Sugars: 5g

Chicken and Zucchini Stir-Fry

Preparation Time: 10 minutes
Cooking Time: 10 minutes
Portions: 1
Ingredients
- ½ cup sliced chicken breast
- ½ zucchini, sliced
- ¼ cup shredded carrots
- 1 tablespoon olive oil
- 1 tablespoon gluten-free soy sauce
- 1 teaspoon sesame seeds

Instructions
1. Heat olive oil in a skillet over medium heat.
2. Add the sliced chicken and cook until browned, about 5-7 minutes.
3. Add zucchini and shredded carrots, cooking for an additional 3-4 minutes.
4. Stir in the gluten-free soy sauce and sesame seeds.
5. Serve warm.

Nutritional Values:
Calories: 320 | Protein: 26g | Fat: 16g | Carbohydrates: 12g | Fiber: 3g | Sugars: 3g

Garlic-Infused Shrimp and Zucchini

Preparation Time: 10 minutes
Cooking Time: 10 minutes
Portions: 1
Ingredients
- ½ cup shrimp, peeled and deveined
- ½ zucchini, sliced
- 1 tablespoon garlic-infused oil
- 1 teaspoon lemon juice
- Salt and pepper to taste
- 1 tablespoon fresh parsley, chopped

Instructions
1. Preheat the oven to 400°F (200°C).
2. Place shrimp and zucchini on a sheet pan.
3. Drizzle with garlic-infused oil and lemon juice.
4. Add salt, pepper, and chopped parsley.
5. Bake for 10 minutes or until shrimp are fully cooked.
6. Serve warm.

Nutritional Values:
Calories: 260 | Protein: 22g | Fat: 14g | Carbohydrates: 6g | Fiber: 2g | Sugars: 2g

Honey Mustard Chicken with Sweet Potatoes

Preparation Time: 10 minutes
Cooking Time: 25 minutes
Portions: 1
Ingredients
- 1 chicken breast
- ½ sweet potato, diced
- 1 tablespoon honey
- 1 tablespoon Dijon mustard
- 1 tablespoon olive oil
- Salt to taste

Instructions
1. Preheat the oven to 400°F (200°C).
2. Mix honey, mustard, and olive oil together to form a glaze.
3. Place the chicken and diced sweet potatoes on a baking sheet and brush the chicken with the glaze.
4. Roast for 25 minutes or until the chicken is cooked through and sweet potatoes are tender.
5. Serve warm.

Nutritional Values:
Calories: 340 | Protein: 26g | Fat: 14g | Carbohydrates: 28g | Fiber: 4g | Sugars: 10g

Lemon Herb Chicken Pasta

Preparation Time: 10 minutes
Cooking Time: 15 minutes
Portions: 1
Ingredients
- 1 cup gluten-free pasta
- ½ cup cooked chicken breast, sliced
- 1 tablespoon lemon juice
- 1 tablespoon olive oil
- 1 tablespoon fresh parsley, chopped
- Salt to taste

Instructions
1. Cook the pasta according to package instructions.
2. In a pan, heat olive oil and toss in the chicken slices, lemon juice, and parsley.
3. Add the cooked pasta to the pan and stir to combine.
4. Serve warm.

Nutritional Values:
Calories: 400 | Protein: 26g | Fat: 12g | Carbohydrates: 50g | Fiber: 4g | Sugars: 1g

Lemon Herb Tilapia and Broccoli

Preparation Time: 10 minutes
Cooking Time: 20 minutes
Portions: 1
Ingredients
- 1 tilapia fillet
- 1 cup broccoli florets
- 1 tablespoon olive oil
- 1 teaspoon lemon zest
- 1 tablespoon fresh parsley, chopped
- Salt to taste

Instructions
1. Preheat the oven to 400°F (200°C).
2. Place tilapia fillet and broccoli on a sheet pan.
3. Drizzle with olive oil, sprinkle with lemon zest, parsley, and salt.
4. Bake for 20 minutes or until the tilapia is fully cooked and broccoli is tender.
5. Serve warm.

Nutritional Values:
Calories: 290 | Protein: 24g | Fat: 14g | Carbohydrates: 10g | Fiber: 5g | Sugars: 2g

Lentil and Spinach Stew

Preparation Time: 10 minutes
Cooking Time: 25 minutes
Portions: 1
Ingredients
- ½ cup lentils
- 1 cup spinach
- ¼ cup diced carrots
- 1 cup gluten-free vegetable broth
- 1 tablespoon olive oil
- 1 teaspoon thyme

Instructions
1. Heat olive oil in a pot over medium heat.
2. Add diced carrots and cook for 2-3 minutes.
3. Stir in lentils and vegetable broth and bring to a boil.
4. Reduce heat and simmer for 20 minutes until lentils are tender.
5. Add spinach and thyme, cooking for another 2 minutes.
6. Serve warm.

Nutritional Values:
Calories: 280 | Protein: 14g | Fat: 8g | Carbohydrates: 38g | Fiber: 12g | Sugars: 5g

One-Pot Lemon Chicken and Rice

Preparation Time: 10 minutes
Cooking Time: 25 minutes
Portions: 1
Ingredients
- ½ cup chicken breast, sliced
- ½ cup white rice (uncooked)
- 1 cup spinach
- 1 tablespoon olive oil
- 1 teaspoon lemon juice
- 1 tablespoon garlic-infused oil

Instructions
1. Heat olive oil in a pot over medium heat.
2. Add chicken slices and cook until browned, about 5 minutes.
3. Stir in the uncooked rice and garlic-infused oil and cook for 1 minute.
4. Add 1 cup of water, cover, and simmer for 15-20 minutes until the rice is cooked.
5. Stir in spinach and lemon juice and cook for another 2 minutes.
6. Serve warm.

Nutritional Values:
Calories: 350 | Protein: 24g | Fat: 12g | Carbohydrates: 38g | Fiber: 3g | Sugars: 1g

Pasta with Roasted Red Pepper Sauce

Preparation Time: 10 minutes
Cooking Time: 20 minutes
Portions: 1
Ingredients
- 1 cup gluten-free pasta
- 1 roasted red pepper, blended
- 2 tablespoons lactose-free cream
- 1 tablespoon olive oil
- Salt and pepper to taste

Instructions
1. Cook the pasta according to package instructions.
2. In a pan, heat olive oil and add the blended roasted red pepper.
3. Stir in the lactose-free cream, salt, and pepper.
4. Toss the cooked pasta with the sauce and serve warm.

Nutritional Values:
Calories: 380 | Protein: 8g | Fat: 14g | Carbohydrates: 56g | Fiber: 5g | Sugars: 6g

Peanut Noodles

Preparation Time: 5 minutes
Cooking Time: 10 minutes
Portions: 1

Ingredients
- 1 cup gluten-free noodles
- 1 tablespoon peanut butter (unsweetened)
- 1 tablespoon gluten-free soy sauce
- 1 teaspoon lime juice
- 1 cup spinach
- ¼ cup shredded carrots

Instructions
1. Cook the noodles according to package instructions.
2. In a bowl, mix peanut butter, soy sauce, and lime juice to make a sauce.
3. Toss the noodles with the sauce, spinach, and shredded carrots.
4. Serve warm or cold.

Nutritional Values:
Calories: 380 | Protein: 12g | Fat: 18g | Carbohydrates: 46g | Fiber: 6g | Sugars: 4g

Pesto Rice with Grilled Chicken

Preparation Time: 10 minutes
Cooking Time: 20 minutes
Portions: 1

Ingredients
- ½ cup cooked brown rice
- ½ cup grilled chicken breast, sliced
- 2 tablespoons lactose-free Parmesan cheese
- 1 tablespoon olive oil
- ¼ cup fresh basil
- 1 tablespoon pine nuts

Instructions
1. In a food processor, blend the fresh basil, pine nuts, olive oil, and lactose-free Parmesan until smooth to make the pesto.
2. In a serving bowl, combine the cooked brown rice with the sliced grilled chicken.
3. Add the freshly made pesto to the rice and chicken, mixing thoroughly.
4. Toss everything until well coated with the pesto.
5. Serve warm and enjoy.

Nutritional Values:
Calories: 400 | Protein: 28g | Fat: 16g | Carbohydrates: 38g | Fiber: 4g | Sugars: 2g

Pork and Potato Hash

Preparation Time: 10 minutes
Cooking Time: 20 minutes
Portions: 1
Ingredients
- ½ cup ground pork
- ½ cup diced potatoes
- 1 cup spinach
- 1 tablespoon olive oil
- 1 teaspoon thyme
- Salt to taste

Instructions
1. Heat olive oil in a skillet over medium heat.
2. Add diced potatoes and cook for 10-12 minutes until tender.
3. Stir in ground pork and cook until browned, about 5-7 minutes.
4. Add spinach, thyme, and salt, cooking until the spinach wilts.
5. Serve warm.

Nutritional Values:
Calories: 380 | Protein: 20g | Fat: 24g | Carbohydrates: 22g | Fiber: 4g | Sugars: 2g

Rice with Tomato Basil Sauce

Preparation Time: 10 minutes
Cooking Time: 15 minutes
Portions: 1
Ingredients
- ½ cup cooked white rice
- ½ cup canned tomatoes
- 1 tablespoon olive oil
- 2 tablespoons fresh basil, chopped
- Salt to taste
- 2 tablespoons lactose-free Parmesan cheese

Instructions
1. In a pan, heat the olive oil over medium heat, then sauté the canned tomatoes and chopped basil for 5 minutes until fragrant.
2. In a serving bowl, mix the cooked white rice with the tomato basil sauce.
3. Top the rice with lactose-free Parmesan cheese.
4. Season with salt to taste.
5. Serve warm and enjoy.

Nutritional Values:
Calories: 320 | Protein: 8g | Fat: 14g | Carbohydrates: 40g | Fiber: 4g | Sugars: 4g

Roasted Chicken Sausage with Bell Peppers

Preparation Time: 10 minutes
Cooking Time: 20 minutes
Portions: 1
Ingredients
- 1 chicken sausage
- 1 bell pepper, sliced
- 1 tablespoon olive oil
- ½ teaspoon thyme
- Salt and pepper to taste

Instructions
1. Preheat the oven to 400°F (200°C).
2. Place chicken sausage and bell pepper slices on a sheet pan.
3. Drizzle with olive oil, sprinkle with thyme, salt, and pepper.
4. Bake for 20 minutes or until sausage is fully cooked and peppers are tender.
5. Serve warm.

Nutritional Values:
Calories: 280 | Protein: 16g | Fat: 18g | Carbohydrates: 10g | Fiber: 3g | Sugars: 5g

Roasted Tofu with Brussels Sprouts

Preparation Time: 10 minutes
Cooking Time: 20 minutes
Portions: 1
Ingredients
1. ½ cup firm tofu, cubed
2. ½ cup Brussels sprouts, halved
3. 1 tablespoon olive oil
4. 1 tablespoon balsamic vinegar
5. Salt and pepper to taste

Instructions
1. Preheat the oven to 400°F (200°C).
2. Place tofu cubes and Brussels sprouts on a sheet pan.
3. Drizzle with olive oil and balsamic vinegar.
4. Add salt and pepper.
5. Bake for 20 minutes or until the Brussels sprouts are tender and tofu is golden brown.
6. Serve warm.

Nutritional Values:
Calories: 280 | Protein: 12g | Fat: 18g | Carbohydrates: 18g | Fiber: 5g | Sugars: 4g

Salmon and Rice Bowl

Preparation Time: 10 minutes
Cooking Time: 15 minutes
Portions: 1
Ingredients
- 1 salmon fillet
- ½ cup cooked white rice
- 1 cup spinach
- 1 tablespoon olive oil
- 1 teaspoon lemon juice
- Salt to taste

Instructions
1. Heat olive oil in a skillet over medium heat.
2. Add the salmon fillet and cook for 4-5 minutes per side until cooked through.
3. In a bowl, layer the cooked rice and spinach.
4. Place the cooked salmon on top, drizzle with lemon juice, and season with salt.
5. Serve warm.

Nutritional Values:
Calories: 420 | Protein: 28g | Fat: 20g | Carbohydrates: 30g | Fiber: 3g | Sugars: 1g

Shrimp and Lemon Risotto

Preparation Time: 10 minutes
Cooking Time: 25 minutes
Portions: 1
Ingredients
- ½ cup Arborio rice
- ½ cup shrimp
- 1 tablespoon lemon juice
- 1 tablespoon lactose-free butter
- 1 tablespoon olive oil
- 1 cup spinach

Instructions
1. In a pan, heat the olive oil and lactose-free butter over medium heat. Add the Arborio rice and cook for 2 minutes, stirring constantly.
2. Gradually add water (or vegetable broth) to the rice, a little at a time, stirring continuously until the rice absorbs the liquid and becomes tender, about 15-20 minutes.
3. Once the rice is cooked, stir in the shrimp, lemon juice, and spinach.
4. Continue cooking until the shrimp are fully cooked and the spinach is wilted.
5. Serve warm and enjoy.

Nutritional Values:
Calories: 380 | Protein: 18g | Fat: 14g | Carbohydrates: 46g | Fiber: 4g | Sugars: 1g

Tofu and Vegetable Stir-Fry

Preparation Time: 10 minutes
Cooking Time: 10 minutes
Portions: 1
Ingredients
- ½ cup firm tofu, cubed
- ½ zucchini, sliced
- ¼ cup shredded carrots
- 1 cup spinach
- 1 tablespoon olive oil
- 1 tablespoon gluten-free soy sauce

Instructions
1. Heat olive oil in a skillet over medium heat.
2. Add tofu cubes and cook for 3-4 minutes until golden brown.
3. Stir in zucchini, carrots, and spinach, cooking for an additional 3-4 minutes.
4. Add gluten-free soy sauce and stir well.
5. Serve warm.

Nutritional Values:
Calories: 290 | Protein: 14g | Fat: 16g | Carbohydrates: 24g | Fiber: 5g | Sugars: 3g

Turkey and Bell Pepper Skillet

Preparation Time: 10 minutes
Cooking Time: 15 minutes
Portions: 1
Ingredients
- ½ cup ground turkey
- ½ bell pepper, sliced
- 1 cup spinach
- 1 tablespoon olive oil
- ½ teaspoon cumin
- Salt to taste

Instructions
1. Heat olive oil in a skillet over medium heat.
2. Add ground turkey and cook until browned, about 5-7 minutes.
3. Stir in bell pepper slices and cook for another 3-4 minutes.
4. Add spinach, cumin, and salt, cooking until the spinach wilts.
5. Serve warm.

Nutritional Values:
Calories: 320 | Protein: 24g | Fat: 16g | Carbohydrates: 14g | Fiber: 4g | Sugars: 3g

Turkey and Zucchini Meatballs with Roasted Potatoes

Preparation Time: 10 minutes
Cooking Time: 25 minutes
Portions: 1

Ingredients
- ½ cup ground turkey
- ½ zucchini, grated
- ½ cup potatoes, diced
- 1 tablespoon olive oil
- ½ teaspoon thyme
- Salt to taste

Instructions
1. Preheat the oven to 400°F (200°C).
2. Mix ground turkey with grated zucchini, form into meatballs.
3. Place meatballs and diced potatoes on a sheet pan.
4. Drizzle with olive oil, sprinkle with thyme and salt.
5. Bake for 25 minutes or until the meatballs are fully cooked and potatoes are tender.
6. Serve warm.

Nutritional Values:
Calories: 320 | Protein: 24g | Fat: 14g | Carbohydrates: 24g | Fiber: 4g | Sugars: 2g

Chapter 11 (25 recipes): Snacks and On-the-Go Solutions

Almond Butter Rice Cakes

Preparation Time: 5 minutes
Cooking Time: None
Portions: 1
Ingredients
- 2 rice cakes
- 1 tablespoon almond butter
- ½ unripe banana, sliced
- 1 teaspoon chia seeds

Instructions
1. Spread the almond butter evenly over both rice cakes.
2. Place the banana slices on top of the almond butter.
3. Sprinkle chia seeds over the banana slices.
4. Serve immediately and enjoy.

Nutritional Values:
Calories: 220 | Protein: 6g | Fat: 10g | Carbohydrates: 30g | Fiber: 4g | Sugars: 5g

Banana Coconut Chia Pudding

Preparation Time: 5 minutes
Cooking Time: 0 minutes (overnight chill)
Portions: 1
Ingredients:
- 1/2 ripe banana, mashed
- 2 tbsp chia seeds
- 1/2 cup lactose-free coconut milk
- 1 tsp maple syrup (optional)
- 1 tbsp shredded coconut (unsweetened)

Instructions:
1. In a bowl, mash the banana.
2. Add chia seeds, coconut milk, maple syrup (if using), and shredded coconut. Stir to combine.
3. Cover and refrigerate overnight or for at least 4 hours until it thickens.
4. Serve chilled, topped with additional coconut if desired.

Nutritional Values:
Calories: 210 | Protein: 4g | Fat: 12g | Carbs: 23g | Fiber: 9g

Banana Oat Muffins

Preparation Time: 10 minutes
Cooking Time: 20 minutes
Portions: 1
Ingredients
- ½ cup gluten-free oats
- 1 unripe banana, mashed
- ¼ cup lactose-free Greek yogurt
- 1 tablespoon maple syrup
- ½ teaspoon cinnamon
- ½ teaspoon baking powder

Instructions
1. Preheat the oven to 350°F (175°C).
2. In a bowl, mix the mashed banana, Greek yogurt, maple syrup, and cinnamon.
3. Stir in the oats and baking powder until combined.
4. Pour the mixture into a muffin tin and bake for 20 minutes.
5. Let cool before serving.

Nutritional Values:
Calories: 200 | Protein: 6g | Fat: 4g | Carbohydrates: 36g | Fiber: 4g | Sugars: 12g

Blueberry Almond Granola Bars

Preparation Time: 10 minutes
Cooking Time: 15 minutes
Portions: 1
Ingredients
- ¼ cup gluten-free oats
- 2 tablespoons dried blueberries (low-FODMAP portion)
- 2 tablespoons almond butter
- 1 tablespoon maple syrup
- 1 teaspoon chia seeds
- ½ teaspoon cinnamon

Instructions
1. Preheat the oven to 350°F (175°C).
2. In a bowl, mix all ingredients until combined.
3. Press the mixture into a small baking dish and bake for 15 minutes.
4. Let cool before cutting into bars.

Nutritional Values:
Calories: 210 | Protein: 6g | Fat: 10g | Carbohydrates: 28g | Fiber: 4g | Sugars: 12g

Blueberry Almond Mug Cake

Preparation Time: 5 minutes
Cooking Time: 2 minutes
Portions: 1
Ingredients:
- 1/4 cup almond flour
- 1 tbsp maple syrup
- 1/4 tsp baking powder
- 1/4 tsp vanilla extract
- 1 tbsp fresh blueberries
- 1 egg (or egg substitute)

Instructions:
1. In a microwave-safe mug, combine almond flour, maple syrup, baking powder, and vanilla extract.
2. Crack the egg into the mixture and whisk until smooth.
3. Gently fold in the blueberries.
4. Microwave on high for 1.5 to 2 minutes or until the cake is set.
5. Let cool for a minute before enjoying.

Nutritional Values:
Calories: 220 | Protein: 8g | Fat: 15g | Carbs: 14g | Fiber: 4g

Blueberry Chia Pudding

Preparation Time: 5 minutes
Cooking Time: None (chill for at least 2 hours)
Portions: 1
Ingredients
- 2 tablespoons chia seeds
- ½ cup almond milk
- ¼ cup fresh blueberries
- 1 teaspoon maple syrup

Instructions
1. In a small jar, mix the chia seeds, almond milk, and maple syrup until well combined.
2. Stir the mixture again after a few minutes to prevent clumping.
3. Refrigerate for at least 2 hours or overnight to allow the pudding to set.
4. Once set, top with fresh blueberries.
5. Serve chilled and enjoy.

Nutritional Values:
Calories: 150 | Protein: 4g | Fat: 8g | Carbohydrates: 18g | Fiber: 6g | Sugars: 7g

Cinnamon Walnut Oat Bars

Preparation Time: 10 minutes
Cooking Time: 15 minutes
Portions: 1
Ingredients
- ¼ cup gluten-free oats
- 2 tablespoons chopped walnuts
- 1 teaspoon cinnamon
- 1 tablespoon maple syrup
- 1 tablespoon lactose-free butter
- 1 teaspoon chia seeds

Instructions
1. Preheat the oven to 350°F (175°C).
2. In a bowl, mix all ingredients until combined.
3. Press into a small baking dish and bake for 15 minutes.
4. Let cool before cutting into bars.

Nutritional Values:
Calories: 200 | Protein: 4g | Fat: 12g | Carbohydrates: 22g | Fiber: 3g | Sugars: 8g

Coconut Almond Energy Balls

Preparation Time: 10 minutes
Cooking Time: None
Portions: 1
Ingredients
- ¼ cup shredded coconut
- 1 tablespoon almond butter
- 2 tablespoons gluten-free oats
- 1 teaspoon chia seeds
- 1 teaspoon maple syrup
- ¼ teaspoon vanilla extract

Instructions
1. In a bowl, combine the shredded coconut, almond butter, gluten-free oats, chia seeds, maple syrup, and vanilla extract until a sticky dough forms.
2. Using your hands, roll the mixture into small, bite-sized balls.
3. Place the energy balls on a plate or tray and refrigerate for 30 minutes to firm up.
4. Once chilled, serve and enjoy.
5. Store any leftovers in the refrigerator for later.

Nutritional Values:
Calories: 150 | Protein: 4g | Fat: 10g | Carbohydrates: 12g | Fiber: 3g | Sugars: 5g

Cucumber and Turkey Roll-Ups

Preparation Time: 5 minutes
Cooking Time: None
Portions: 1
Ingredients
- 4 slices turkey
- ½ cucumber, sliced
- 2 tablespoons lactose-free cream cheese
- 1 cup spinach

Instructions
1. Spread the lactose-free cream cheese evenly over each turkey slice.
2. Place cucumber slices and a few spinach leaves on top of the cream cheese.
3. Gently roll each turkey slice around the filling to create roll-ups.
4. Arrange on a plate and serve immediately.
5. Enjoy as a light snack or appetizer.

Nutritional Values:
Calories: 180 | Protein: 16g | Fat: 8g | Carbohydrates: 8g | Fiber: 2g | Sugars: 2g

Dark Chocolate Almond Energy Bars

Preparation Time: 10 minutes
Cooking Time: 15 minutes
Portions: 1
Ingredients
- ¼ cup chopped almonds
- 2 tablespoons lactose-free dark chocolate, melted
- 2 tablespoons gluten-free oats
- 1 tablespoon coconut oil
- 1 teaspoon chia seeds
- 1 tablespoon maple syrup

Instructions
1. Preheat the oven to 350°F (175°C).
2. Mix all ingredients in a bowl.
3. Press the mixture into a small baking dish and bake for 15 minutes.
4. Let cool before cutting into bars.

Nutritional Values:
Calories: 230 | Protein: 6g | Fat: 16g | Carbohydrates: 18g | Fiber: 4g | Sugars: 8g

Dark Chocolate Dipped Strawberries

Preparation Time: 5 minutes
Cooking Time: 5 minutes
Portions: 1
Ingredients:
- 6 large strawberries
- 1/4 cup dark chocolate chips (low-FODMAP approved)
- 1/2 tsp coconut oil

Instructions:
1. Melt dark chocolate chips and coconut oil in a microwave-safe bowl, heating in 15-second intervals and stirring until smooth.
2. Dip each strawberry into the melted chocolate, coating halfway.
3. Place the strawberries on a parchment-lined tray and let them cool until the chocolate sets (refrigerate for faster results).
4. Serve chilled or at room temperature.

Nutritional Values:
Calories: 180 | Protein: 2g | Fat: 12g | Carbs: 19g | Fiber: 5g

Egg Salad Lettuce Cups

Preparation Time: 10 minutes
Cooking Time: None
Portions: 1
Ingredients
- 2 hard-boiled eggs, chopped
- 1 tablespoon lactose-free mayonnaise
- 1 teaspoon Dijon mustard
- 3 romaine lettuce leaves

Instructions
1. In a bowl, mix the chopped hard-boiled eggs, lactose-free mayonnaise, and Dijon mustard until well combined.
2. Spoon the egg salad mixture evenly into the romaine lettuce leaves, forming lettuce cups.
3. Serve immediately and enjoy as a light, refreshing meal or snack.

Nutritional Values:
Calories: 240 | Protein: 12g | Fat: 18g | Carbohydrates: 2g | Fiber: 1g | Sugars: 0g

Gluten-Free Crackers with Avocado Slices

Preparation Time: 5 minutes
Cooking Time: None
Portions: 1
Ingredients
- 4 gluten-free crackers
- ½ avocado, sliced
- 1 teaspoon lemon juice
- 1 teaspoon olive oil
- Salt to taste

Instructions
1. Arrange the avocado slices on the crackers.
2. Drizzle with lemon juice and olive oil, and sprinkle with salt.
3. Serve immediately.

Nutritional Values:
Calories: 200 | Protein: 3g | Fat: 14g | Carbohydrates: 16g | Fiber: 6g | Sugars: 1g

Hard-Boiled Eggs with Cherry Tomatoes

Preparation Time: 10 minutes
Cooking Time: 10 minutes
Portions: 1
Ingredients
- 2 hard-boiled eggs
- ½ cup cherry tomatoes, halved
- ¼ cup spinach
- 1 teaspoon olive oil
- Salt to taste

Instructions
1. Hard-boil the eggs and slice them in half.
2. Toss cherry tomatoes and spinach in olive oil and a pinch of salt.
3. Serve the eggs with the tomato-spinach mixture.

Nutritional Values:
Calories: 180 | Protein: 12g | Fat: 12g | Carbohydrates: 6g | Fiber: 2g | Sugars: 4g

Honey Almond Nut Mix

Preparation Time: 5 minutes
Cooking Time: None
Portions: 1
Ingredients
- 2 tablespoons almonds
- 1 tablespoon pumpkin seeds
- 1 tablespoon sunflower seeds
- 1 teaspoon coconut oil
- 1 teaspoon honey
- Pinch of sea salt

Instructions
1. In a bowl, combine the almonds, pumpkin seeds, sunflower seeds, coconut oil, honey, and a pinch of sea salt.
2. Stir well to ensure everything is evenly coated.
3. Serve immediately as a snack or store in an airtight container for later.
4. Enjoy as a quick, energy-boosting treat!

Nutritional Values:
Calories: 180 | Protein: 5g | Fat: 14g | Carbohydrates: 12g | Fiber: 3g | Sugars: 6g

Kale Chips

Preparation Time: 5 minutes
Cooking Time: 15 minutes
Portions: 1
Ingredients
- 1 cup kale, torn into bite-sized pieces
- 1 tablespoon olive oil
- Salt and pepper to taste

Instructions
1. Preheat the oven to 350°F (175°C).
2. Toss kale with olive oil, salt, and pepper.
3. Spread on a baking sheet and bake for 12-15 minutes until crispy.
4. Serve immediately.

Nutritional Values:
Calories: 80 | Protein: 2g | Fat: 7g | Carbohydrates: 5g | Fiber: 1g | Sugars: 1g

Lactose-Free Greek Yogurt Parfait

Preparation Time: 5 minutes
Cooking Time: None
Portions: 1
Ingredients
- ½ cup lactose-free Greek yogurt
- ¼ cup strawberries, sliced
- 2 tablespoons gluten-free granola
- 1 teaspoon chia seeds

Instructions
1. In a serving bowl, layer the lactose-free Greek yogurt, followed by the sliced strawberries, and then the gluten-free granola.
2. Sprinkle the chia seeds evenly on top.
3. Serve immediately and enjoy this refreshing and nutritious parfait.

Nutritional Values:
Calories: 210 | Protein: 10g | Fat: 8g | Carbohydrates: 26g | Fiber: 4g | Sugars: 8g

Peanut Butter and Celery Sticks

Preparation Time: 5 minutes
Cooking Time: None
Portions: 1
Ingredients
- 2 celery sticks
- 1 tablespoon peanut butter
- 1 teaspoon chia seeds

Instructions
1. Spread peanut butter along the length of the celery sticks.
2. Sprinkle with chia seeds.
3. Serve immediately.

Nutritional Values:
Calories: 140 | Protein: 5g | Fat: 10g | Carbohydrates: 9g | Fiber: 4g | Sugars: 2g

Peanut Butter Chocolate Chip Cookies (Gluten-Free)

Preparation Time: 5 minutes
Cooking Time: 10 minutes
Portions: 1 (4 small cookies)
Ingredients:
- 2 tbsp peanut butter (natural, unsweetened)
- 2 tbsp gluten-free oat flour
- 1 tbsp dark chocolate chips (low-FODMAP approved)
- 1 tbsp maple syrup
- 1/4 tsp baking soda

Instructions:
1. Preheat oven to 350°F (180°C).
2. In a bowl, mix peanut butter, oat flour, baking soda, and maple syrup until combined.
3. Fold in dark chocolate chips.
4. Drop spoonfuls of dough onto a parchment-lined baking sheet.
5. Bake for 8-10 minutes or until lightly golden. Let cool before serving.

Nutritional Values:
Calories: 210 | Protein: 6g | Fat: 12g | Carbs: 22g | Fiber: 4g

Peanut Butter Oat Energy Bites

Preparation Time: 10 minutes
Cooking Time: None (chill for 30 minutes)
Portions: 1
Ingredients
- ¼ cup gluten-free oats
- 1 tablespoon peanut butter
- 1 teaspoon chia seeds
- 1 teaspoon maple syrup

Instructions
1. In a bowl, combine the gluten-free oats, peanut butter, chia seeds, and maple syrup, mixing until a sticky dough forms.
2. Roll the mixture into small bite-sized balls using your hands.
3. Place the energy bites on a plate and refrigerate for 30 minutes to firm up.
4. Once chilled, serve and enjoy.
5. Store any leftovers in the refrigerator for later.

Nutritional Values:
Calories: 150 | Protein: 4g | Fat: 8g | Carbohydrates: 18g | Fiber: 3g | Sugars: 5g

Raspberry Coconut Macaroons

Preparation Time: 5 minutes
Cooking Time: 10 minutes
Portions: 1 (4 small macaroons)
Ingredients:
- 1/2 cup shredded coconut (unsweetened)
- 1 tbsp maple syrup
- 1 egg white
- 1 tbsp fresh raspberries, mashed

Instructions:
1. Preheat oven to 350°F (180°C).
2. In a bowl, mix shredded coconut, maple syrup, and mashed raspberries.
3. Whisk the egg white until frothy and fold into the coconut mixture.
4. Form small balls and place them on a parchment-lined baking sheet.
5. Bake for 10-12 minutes or until golden brown. Let cool before serving.

Nutritional Values:
Calories: 160 | Protein: 3g | Fat: 10g | Carbs: 15g | Fiber: 5g

Roasted Pumpkin Seeds

Preparation Time: 5 minutes
Cooking Time: 20 minutes
Portions: 1
Ingredients
- ¼ cup pumpkin seeds
- 1 teaspoon olive oil
- Salt and paprika to taste

Instructions
1. Preheat the oven to 350°F (175°C).
2. Toss pumpkin seeds with olive oil, salt, and paprika.
3. Spread on a baking sheet and roast for 15-20 minutes, stirring halfway through.
4. Serve warm or cool.

Nutritional Values:
Calories: 130 | Protein: 5g | Fat: 11g | Carbohydrates: 5g | Fiber: 2g | Sugars: 0g

Turkey and Swiss Lettuce Wraps

Preparation Time: 5 minutes
Cooking Time: None
Portions: 1

Ingredients
- 2 slices turkey
- 1 slice lactose-free Swiss cheese
- 2 romaine lettuce leaves
- 1 teaspoon mustard
- 1 teaspoon olive oil

Instructions
1. Lay the romaine lettuce leaves flat and place a slice of turkey and lactose-free Swiss cheese on each leaf.
2. Drizzle the mustard and olive oil evenly over the turkey and cheese.
3. Tightly wrap the lettuce around the fillings to form wraps.
4. Serve immediately and enjoy as a light, fresh snack or meal.

Nutritional Values:
Calories: 150 | Protein: 15g | Fat: 8g | Carbohydrates: 3g | Fiber: 1g | Sugars: 1g

Zucchini Chips

Preparation Time: 5 minutes
Cooking Time: 25 minutes
Portions: 1

Ingredients
- 1 small zucchini, sliced thinly
- 1 tablespoon olive oil
- Salt to taste
- 1 teaspoon garlic-infused oil

Instructions
1. Preheat the oven to 400°F (200°C).
2. Toss zucchini slices with olive oil, garlic-infused oil, and salt.
3. Spread on a baking sheet and bake for 20-25 minutes until crispy.
4. Serve immediately.

Nutritional Values:
Calories: 90 | Protein: 2g | Fat: 7g | Carbohydrates: 6g | Fiber: 1g | Sugars: 3g

Walnut and Date Energy Bites

Preparation Time: 10 minutes
Cooking Time: None (chill for 30 minutes)
Portions: 1
Ingredients
- 2 tablespoons chopped walnuts
- 2 low-FODMAP portion dates, chopped
- 1 teaspoon chia seeds
- 1 tablespoon shredded coconut
- 1 teaspoon almond butter
- ½ teaspoon cinnamon

Instructions
1. In a bowl, combine the chopped walnuts, chopped dates, chia seeds, shredded coconut, almond butter, and cinnamon. Mix well until a sticky dough forms.
2. Roll the mixture into small bite-sized balls using your hands.
3. Place the energy bites on a plate and refrigerate for 30 minutes to firm up.
4. Once chilled, serve and enjoy.
5. Store any leftovers in an airtight container in the refrigerator for later.

Nutritional Values:
Calories: 200 | Protein: 4g | Fat: 12g | Carbohydrates: 20g | Fiber: 4g | Sugars: 12g

PART IV: EXPERT TIPS AND STRATEGIES FOR SUCCESS

Part IV: Expert Tips and Strategies for Success is where we dive into the practical aspects of living well on a Low-FODMAP diet. By now, you've learned the foundations, explored your triggers, and have started personalizing your meals. But long-term success goes beyond just knowing the basics—it's about finding sustainable strategies that fit into your daily life. In this section, we offer expert insights to help you overcome common challenges, stay motivated, and make this diet feel less restrictive. Whether you're navigating social events or just trying to streamline meal prep, these tips will empower you to stay on track with confidence.

Chapter 14: Managing IBS and Digestive Issues Beyond Diet

Stress Management and Its Role in Gut Health

Stress doesn't just affect your mind; it profoundly influences your digestive system, particularly when dealing with IBS or other gut-related conditions. The gut-brain axis is a critical component in understanding this interaction. This communication network between your gut and brain means that when you're stressed, your brain sends signals to your digestive system, often resulting in a disruption of normal processes. For those managing IBS, this can lead to an exacerbation of symptoms like bloating, abdominal cramps, and irregular bowel movements.

When stress triggers the body's "fight-or-flight" response, your digestion can either slow down or speed up dramatically. This physiological shift happens because your body is prioritizing immediate survival, redirecting energy away from non-essential functions like digestion. For some, this results in constipation as the digestive system slows. For others, it can trigger diarrhea as the system speeds up. The variability depends on individual reactions to stress, but the impact on gut health is undeniable.

Managing stress, therefore, becomes a key strategy for maintaining digestive health, especially when following a Low-FODMAP diet. Mindfulness techniques, such as meditation or yoga, are scientifically shown to reduce stress hormone levels, which can calm the gut. Deep-breathing exercises help activate the body's parasympathetic nervous system—often referred to as the "rest and digest" system—which counteracts the fight-or-flight response, promoting smoother digestion. Light physical activities, such as walking, can also enhance digestion by relieving tension and stimulating gut motility without putting excess pressure on your body.

Incorporating these stress-reducing practices into your daily routine, alongside a personalized Low-FODMAP diet, can offer more control over symptoms. Just as you monitor the foods you eat to identify triggers, regularly assessing your stress levels allows you to take proactive steps in preventing flare-ups. By approaching both diet and stress with intention, you can build a comprehensive plan to manage your digestive health effectively, supporting not just symptom relief but also your overall well-being.

In the long term, recognizing the cyclical relationship between stress and gut health empowers you. When you understand that stress can exacerbate symptoms, you gain the knowledge needed to manage flare-ups more effectively and fine-tune your approach—whether that's adjusting your food intake, increasing relaxation practices, or using a combination of both.

Sleep, Exercise, and Their Impact on Digestion

Sleep and exercise play pivotal roles in digestion and overall gut health, particularly when managing a condition like IBS or following a Low-FODMAP diet. A balanced approach to both can significantly enhance your digestive function, making it easier to manage symptoms and improve your quality of life.

When it comes to sleep, its restorative nature is essential for maintaining healthy digestion. During sleep, the body undergoes critical repair processes, including those affecting the gut lining and overall digestive function. Poor sleep, or insufficient rest, can disrupt these processes and exacerbate symptoms such as bloating, cramps, and irregular bowel movements. Studies show that sleep deprivation can increase the perception of pain and discomfort, making digestive issues feel more severe. It also disrupts the regulation of hunger hormones, potentially leading to overeating or poor food choices, which can further aggravate digestive symptoms.

Exercise, meanwhile, has a dual benefit for both your gut and overall health. Regular physical activity encourages bowel motility, helping prevent constipation and supporting smoother digestion. For individuals with IBS, light to moderate exercise, such as walking or yoga, is often recommended as it can alleviate stress while simultaneously promoting gut function. Exercise helps regulate the digestive system by increasing blood flow to the gastrointestinal tract, which enhances nutrient absorption and waste elimination.

It's important to recognize that while intense physical activity can sometimes exacerbate symptoms in those with sensitive digestion, finding the right balance is key. Engaging in consistent, moderate exercise helps keep the digestive system active and can reduce the occurrence of flare-ups.

Incorporating a routine of consistent, high-quality sleep alongside regular exercise will not only help manage your digestive health but will also enhance the overall benefits of the Low-FODMAP diet. By making these two lifestyles factors a priority, you create a foundation of stability that allows your body to function optimally, supporting digestion, reducing inflammation, and even improving your stress response.

Tracking your sleep patterns and adjusting your physical activity to suit your digestive needs can become as important as monitoring your food intake. By aligning these habits with your Low-FODMAP plan, you take a comprehensive approach to digestive health, making long-term symptom management more achievable and sustainable.

Chapter 15: Navigating Social Events and Dining Out

How to Stick to Low-FODMAP at Restaurants

Sticking to a Low-FODMAP diet at restaurants can be challenging, but with the right approach, it's entirely manageable. The key lies in preparation and communication, both of which empower you to enjoy dining out without compromising your digestive health.

First, research is your ally. Before heading to a restaurant, check their menu online. Look for dishes that are naturally low in FODMAPs, such as grilled meats, fish, salads with suitable dressings, or vegetable-based options. Many restaurants now offer gluten-free or dairy-free dishes, which can often be easier to adapt for a Low-FODMAP meal. If the menu isn't clear, don't hesitate to call ahead and ask if they can accommodate dietary restrictions.

When you arrive, it's important to communicate your needs clearly to your server. Explain that you're following a Low-FODMAP diet, which is essential for managing your digestive health. It's helpful to mention specific triggers like garlic, onion, and high-fructose ingredients, which are common in restaurant dishes. Ask if the kitchen can prepare your food without these ingredients or modify certain dishes to fit your dietary needs. Many chefs are willing to make adjustments, such as using garlic-infused oil instead of raw garlic or offering plain steamed vegetables instead of those cooked in sauces.

Be mindful of potential hidden FODMAPs in sauces, dressings, and marinades. These can often contain high-FODMAP ingredients like honey, wheat, or certain thickeners. Opt for simple, whole-food preparations like grilled meats, steamed vegetables, or a plain baked potato, and request dressings or sauces on the side so you can control your intake.

Another tip is to stick to dishes with ingredients you know are safe for you. For example, choose salads with leafy greens, cucumbers, and tomatoes, paired with a simple olive oil and lemon dressing. Grain-based dishes like quinoa or rice can also be safe, provided they aren't cooked with high-FODMAP broths or additives.

Desserts are often trickier, as many contain high-FODMAP ingredients like lactose, fructose, or wheat. If you're craving something sweet, fresh fruit or a simple fruit sorbet (without added sweeteners) can be a safe bet. Alternatively, you can skip dessert and treat yourself to a low-FODMAP snack when you get home.

Ultimately, flexibility is key. If you find that a restaurant doesn't offer many Low-FODMAP options, it's perfectly okay to bring along a small snack, such as a Low-FODMAP energy bar, to enjoy afterward.

By preparing in advance and advocating for your needs, you can confidently stick to your Low-FODMAP diet while still enjoying the experience of dining out.

Dining out on a Low-FODMAP diet may require some adjustments, but with practice, you'll find it easier to navigate restaurant menus, communicate your needs effectively, and enjoy meals that support your digestive health.

Tips for Traveling While Following the Diet

Traveling while following a Low-FODMAP diet requires thoughtful planning, but it can be done smoothly with the right strategies in place. Preparation is key, as traveling often means facing unpredictable food options, whether at airports, on planes, or in unfamiliar restaurants. To stay on track, you can take several steps to maintain your digestive health while away from home.

First, always pack a variety of Low-FODMAP snacks to have on hand. Items such as rice cakes, lactose-free yogurt, hard-boiled eggs, or homemade Low-FODMAP energy bars can be lifesavers when you're on the move and don't have access to safe meal options. Snacks like these can keep you satisfied and prevent you from having to compromise with potentially high-FODMAP foods in a pinch. It's also wise to bring some easy-to-carry foods like almond butter packets, gluten-free crackers, or dried low-FODMAP fruits like banana chips.

When traveling by air, airports and airplanes often offer limited food choices, many of which may contain hidden FODMAPs. If possible, pack your own meal for the flight. For example, a salad with Low-FODMAP vegetables and a protein like grilled chicken or tuna, or even a sandwich made with gluten-free bread, will help ensure you stick to your diet and avoid discomfort.

Staying in accommodations with a small kitchen or at least a refrigerator can be a huge help when traveling. This allows you to prepare or store your own meals and snacks, reducing reliance on eating out for every meal. You can visit local grocery stores to buy fresh, Low-FODMAP ingredients such as fruits, vegetables, and gluten-free products to make quick meals in your room. This not only keeps you in control of your diet but can also help save money.

When dining out while traveling, apply the same strategies you use at home—research restaurants ahead of time and review their menus for Low-FODMAP options. Don't hesitate to ask the staff about ingredients or make special requests for your meals. International travel can be a bit more challenging, especially if there are language barriers. In such cases, it may help to carry a card that explains your dietary needs in the local language. These cards can help you clearly communicate your food restrictions and avoid ingredients that could trigger symptoms.

Finally, be flexible and patient with yourself. Travel inevitably brings new experiences, and while it's important to stick to your Low-FODMAP plan as much as possible, it's also essential to enjoy the journey. If you find yourself in a situation where you need to make the best of what's available, do so mindfully. If necessary, you can reset your system after your trip and continue to manage your digestive health with greater ease.

With a bit of planning and awareness, traveling while on the Low-FODMAP diet can be an enjoyable and stress-free experience.

Chapter 16: Supplements and Additional Support

Probiotics, Prebiotics, and Their Role in Gut Health

Probiotics and prebiotics play a significant role in maintaining gut health, particularly when managing conditions like IBS or following a Low-FODMAP diet. Both are essential for supporting the balance of healthy gut bacteria, which in turn helps optimize digestion, reduce inflammation, and manage symptoms related to digestive disorders.

Probiotics are live beneficial bacteria that, when consumed in adequate amounts, can help repopulate your gut with good microbes. These friendly bacteria help improve your overall gut environment by balancing the levels of harmful bacteria, which can contribute to symptoms like bloating, diarrhea, or constipation. Some probiotic-rich foods, such as yogurt and kefir, may be Low-FODMAP in small servings, but it's important to choose options that are lactose-free or carefully portioned to avoid triggering symptoms. You can also opt for high-quality probiotic supplements, especially during the elimination phase when your dietary choices may be more limited. A good supplement can help maintain gut diversity and potentially ease discomfort.

Prebiotics, on the other hand, are a form of fiber that acts as food for these beneficial bacteria. Prebiotic fibers aren't digested by your body; instead, they pass through the digestive tract to your colon, where they nourish the good bacteria. While prebiotics are essential for gut health, many foods rich in prebiotics, such as onions, garlic, and certain legumes, are high in FODMAPs and may need to be avoided or reintroduced carefully. During the personalization phase, as you reintroduce foods, you can explore incorporating small amounts of Low-FODMAP prebiotics, like firm bananas, oats, or certain nuts, into your diet.

Together, probiotics and prebiotics form a synergy that can greatly benefit your digestive health. Probiotics bring in new bacteria, while prebiotics support the growth and activity of those beneficial bacteria. As you navigate through the phases of the Low-FODMAP diet, balancing both of these elements becomes vital in restoring and maintaining a healthy gut. You can work with your healthcare provider to ensure you're getting enough of both in ways that align with your unique triggers and tolerance levels. This balance not only helps manage IBS symptoms but also supports your long-term digestive well-being.

By prioritizing the integration of both probiotics and prebiotics into your routine, you take a proactive approach to cultivating a gut environment that thrives and keeps your symptoms under control. Regularly incorporating these elements as part of your Low-FODMAP plan can provide lasting benefits for your overall gut health.

Supplements for IBS Management

Supplements can play a helpful role in managing IBS symptoms, especially when combined with a structured approach like the Low-FODMAP diet. While the foundation of managing IBS lies in diet and lifestyle, certain supplements can support digestive health by targeting specific symptoms such as bloating, cramping, irregular bowel movements, or even stress, which is closely tied to gut function.

One of the most common supplements for IBS management is **fiber supplements**, particularly soluble fiber, which can help regulate bowel movements. If constipation is a key issue, supplements like **psyllium husk** are often recommended because they bulk up stool and promote regularity without being too harsh on the digestive system. However, not all fiber supplements are equal for those with IBS, as some, like inulin, can be high in FODMAPs and may trigger symptoms.

Probiotics are another essential supplement for IBS management. While their effects can vary from person to person, certain strains have been studied for their ability to reduce bloating, gas, and discomfort. The right probiotic supplement can help maintain a healthy balance of gut bacteria, especially if you're still in the process of reintroducing high-FODMAP foods. It's worth discussing specific strains with a healthcare provider, as some may be more effective for IBS than others.

For those who struggle with spasms and cramping, **peppermint oil supplements** have shown promise. Peppermint oil has a relaxing effect on the smooth muscles of the intestines, which can help alleviate abdominal pain and cramping commonly associated with IBS. It's often recommended in enteric-coated capsules to ensure it reaches the intestines without causing heartburn or irritation.

Digestive enzymes can also be beneficial, especially when you're working to reintroduce foods that contain higher FODMAPs, such as lactose or fructans. For instance, **lactase supplements** can help individuals who are sensitive to lactose break down dairy products more easily, while other enzyme blends can target harder-to-digest carbohydrates.

Another supplement to consider is **magnesium**, particularly if constipation is a frequent issue. Magnesium citrate or magnesium oxide can help draw water into the intestines, promoting bowel movements without being too aggressive. However, it's important to use this supplement cautiously, as too much magnesium can lead to diarrhea.

Finally, **stress management supplements** like **L-theanine** or **ashwagandha** can indirectly support digestive health by reducing stress and anxiety, which often worsen IBS symptoms. Since the gut-brain connection plays such a significant role in how your digestive system functions, addressing stress can lead to notable improvements in symptom control.

While supplements can be useful in managing IBS, they should be considered as part of a broader, personalized strategy. It's essential to introduce them gradually and track your body's response, just as you would with reintroducing FODMAP foods. As always, consult with a healthcare professional before starting any new supplement, especially to ensure it aligns with your specific IBS symptoms and overall health plan.

CONCLUSION

As you reach the conclusion of your journey through the Low-FODMAP diet, it's essential to reflect on the progress you've made and the empowerment that comes from truly understanding your body's unique needs. Navigating digestive health, particularly with conditions like IBS, can be challenging, but by now, you've gained the tools and knowledge to manage your symptoms effectively and enjoy a balanced, fulfilling life. The key is to continue listening to your body, adapting your approach as needed, and trusting the process. Your path to long-term digestive wellness doesn't end here—it's just the beginning of a healthier, more informed future.

Recap of the 60-Day Journey

The 60-day journey on the Low-FODMAP diet has been an empowering and transformative experience, providing you with a deeper understanding of your digestive health. In the first phase, you eliminated high-FODMAP foods to reset your system, giving your gut a chance to heal and reduce the burden of common triggers. The reintroduction phase helped you pinpoint specific FODMAP sensitivities, allowing you to clearly identify what your body tolerates well and what it doesn't. Finally, in the personalization phase, you learned how to craft a sustainable, long-term eating plan that supports your unique digestive needs while still enjoying a wide variety of foods. This methodical approach has not only brought relief from symptoms but also given you the tools to confidently manage your gut health moving forward.

You've now gained a solid foundation, equipped with personalized strategies to handle flare-ups, enjoy social events, and navigate the world of food with far less anxiety. Keep in mind that your digestive health is a journey that requires ongoing attention, but the understanding and self-awareness you've developed through this process are invaluable assets in maintaining your well-being.

How to Maintain Long-Term Digestive Health

Maintaining long-term digestive health after completing the 60-day Low-FODMAP journey requires a combination of self-awareness, consistency, and flexibility. Now that you've identified your personal triggers, it's important to integrate that knowledge into your daily life. Continue to monitor your body's reactions to foods, and adjust your diet as needed based on how you feel. It's also key to maintain a diverse and balanced diet that includes a wide variety of low-FODMAP foods, ensuring you get the necessary nutrients to support both digestive and overall health.

Stress management is equally essential—since stress can directly impact your gut, maintaining practices like mindfulness, relaxation exercises, or regular physical activity will help keep symptoms at bay. Stay proactive about hydration, physical movement, and sleep as all these factors significantly contribute to digestive function.

If you experience occasional flare-ups, remember it's not about perfection, but about balance. Use your knowledge from the elimination and reintroduction phases to make temporary adjustments, and then return to your personalized plan. Building a routine that respects both your digestive health, and your overall lifestyle will help you maintain long-term success. You now have the tools to navigate your diet confidently, adapt to changes, and sustain a healthy, happy gut.